RENAL DIET COOKBOOK 2020

The Complete Guide to Manage & Avoid Kidney Disease, Prevent Dialysis. Includes Delicious Recipes, Complete List of Foods to Avoid and Eat

Nancy Peterson

Copyright @ 2020

Table of Content

Introduction..3

Chapter 1: Understanding Kidney Disease 5

Stages of Kidney Disease...6

Connection Between Kidney Disease and Diet.................9

Shopping Tips for Renal Diet...18

Nutrition Label Facts 19

Foods to Avoid on Renal Diet 22

Best Foods to Eat with Kidney Disease 35

Portion Control 49

CHAPTER 2: BREAKFAST RECIPES.................................51

CHAPTER 3: LUNCH RECIPES...87

CHAPTER 4: MAIN DISH RECIPES 93

CHAPTER 5: SIDE DISH RECIPES 122

CHAPTER 6: DINNER RECIPES......................................131

CHAPTER 7: DESSERT RECIPES.....................................143

Conclusion 172

Other Books by the Author 173

Introduction

Kidney disease is quite common and affects about 10 percent of the world's population. Although the kidneys are small, yet they perform several important functions; they help to filter waste products, balance fluids in the body, release hormones that regulate blood pressure, produce urine, amidst other important functions.

Once the kidney is damaged, waste begins to build up in the blood, including waste products from the foods we eat. This is the reason people diagnosed with kidney disease are placed on a special diet called the renal diet, to help heal the kidneys and prevent further damage.

This book is your complete guide to kidney disease and the renal diet. The purpose of writing this loaded book is to ensure that you never have to go through dialysis and to equip you with the right information to prevent the kidney from further damage.

Some of the insights you will benefit from this book include

- Delicious kidney-friendly recipes.

- A clear understanding of kidney disease and the different stages of kidney disease.
- A detailed explanation of the minerals and nutrients you need to avoid or limit while on the renal diet.
- Foods to eat and foods to avoid to succeed with the renal diet
- A detailed explanation of how to read the nutrition label
- Shopping tips for the renal diet
- Understanding of proper portion control for renal diet
- And lots more!

Chapter 1: Understanding Kidney Disease

Studies estimate that about 31 million people in the United States alone have kidney disease, while 1 out of 10 persons in the world have some type of kidney disease. Kidney disease also referred to as renal disease, is a term used for any damage that affects the proper functioning of the kidneys. The human kidneys are heart-shaped organs in the body that performs several vital functions. The kidneys dispose of the waste in the body through our urine, filters the blood, balance minerals, produce hormones and maintain the level of fluid in the body.

Daily, the two kidneys filter approximately 120 - 150 quarts of blood to produce about 1 to 2 quarts of urine, made up of extra fluid and wastes. When the kidneys are healthy, they help to remove water and waste, regulate blood pressure, regulate growth in children, and alert our body to make red blood cells. But once the kidney gets damaged, it becomes unable to carry out these functions properly. Several things can cause harm to the kidney but the most common causes of kidney diseases are high blood pressure and uncontrolled diabetes.

Other causes include HIV infection, heart disease, alcoholism, and hepatitis C virus. When a person's blood pressure and blood sugar level goes beyond normal, it damages the blood vessels in the kidney, causing the kidney not to perform optimally.

Other risk factors for kidney disease include age, gender, genetics, smoking, and obesity. These risk factors increase one's chances of having chronic kidney disease. A patient is diagnosed with chronic kidney disease if the kidneys are not performing their functions and are not able to clean out waste products and toxins from the blood. This chronic disease may take some time to develop or may happen suddenly.

Stages of Kidney Disease

The National Kidney Foundation (NKF) designed a guideline that makes it easy for doctors to identify the different levels of kidney disease. According to the NKF, kidney disease (CKD) has five stages, and the medical practitioner needs to know the stage that a patient is at to be able to provide the best care as each stage has its unique treatment.

For you to properly understand these stages, you need first to know how kidney function is measured. The globally accepted method to measure kidney function is what is referred to as the **Glomerular Filtration Rate (GFR).** A kidney is said to function well if it can clean the human blood and the only way to confirm this is by using the GFR. The GFR is gotten by conducting a blood test that will show the level of creatinine in the blood or serum creatinine; the levels of creatinine increase as the kidney function reduces. To be able to determine the GFR, an equation that includes the serum creatinine along with other factors like gender, race and age, is calculated. Other factors that are considered in this equation are serum albumin, blood urea nitrogen (BUN), and the weight of the patient.

The table below explains the five stages of kidney failure:

Stages of Kidney Disease		
Stages	**Kidney Function/ GFR**	**Description**
Stage 1	>90%	Normal/ High

		Function
Stage 2	60 – 89%	Mildly decreased function
Stage 3	30 – 59%	Mild to moderately decreased function
Stage 4	15 – 29%	Severely decreased function
Stage 5	< 15%	Kidney failure

Below, you will see the five stages of CKD/ kidney disease and the GFR for each of these stages.

- **Stage 1:** normal or high GFR (GFR>90 mL/min)
- **Stage 2:** Mild CKD (GFR is equal to 60 to 89 mL/min)
- **Stage 3A:** Moderate CKD (GFR is equal to 45 to 59 mL/min)
- **Stage 3B:** Moderate CKD (GFR is equal to 30 to 44 mL/ min)
- **Stage 4:** Severe CKD (GFR is equal to 15 to 29 mL/min)

- **Stage 5:** End-stage CKD (GFR is less than 15 mL/min)

Connection Between Kidney Disease and Diet

Diet restrictions depend on the level of damage to the kidney. For example, people with the early stages of kidney disease will have different diet restrictions from persons with end-stage kidney failure or renal disease.

Patients with end-stage kidney failure will require dialysis as well as varying dietary restrictions. These patients undergo dialysis to help filter waste and remove excess water in the body. A large number of those with the end-stage or late stages of kidney failure needs to be on a kidney-friendly diet to prevent the body from accumulating certain chemicals or nutrients in the blood. For patients who have chronic kidney disease, the kidneys will not be able to remove excess phosphorus, potassium, and sodium adequately. Because of this, they have a very high risk of elevated blood levels of these minerals mentioned above.

Most people with advanced kidney disease need to follow a kidney-friendly diet to help reduce the amount of waste in the blood. This diet is what we call the renal diet. The renal diet helps to boost the functions of the kidney while protecting the kidney from further harm.

A renal diet or kidney-friendly diet reduces the amount of potassium and sodium to 2,000 mg daily, while phosphorus is reduced to 1,000 mg daily. A damaged kidney may also experience difficulties with filtering waste products of protein metabolism. It is, therefore, important that people with chronic kidney disease in stages 1 to 4 limit the amount of protein in their diets. However, patients with end-stage renal disease who are undergoing dialysis need to increase their protein intake.

A renal diet is low in protein, phosphorus, and sodium. The diet also lays great emphasis on consuming high-quality protein and reducing your intake of fluids. Some patients may also need to reduce their consumption of calcium and potassium. But like we established already, every individual is different, and their body needs differ; this is why you need to work with a renal dietitian to design a diet that will suit your individual needs.

Although the dietary restrictions differ from person to person, yet, everyone with kidney diseases needs to restrict their consumption of the following nutrients:

Sodium

The body has three major electrolytes, and they are sodium, chloride, and potassium. Electrolytes are responsible for the fluids that go in and out of the cells and tissues in our bodies. Some people believe that sodium and salt are interchangeable. However, salt is actually a compound of chloride and sodium. We may eat foods that contain sodium in other forms other than salt. Processed foods usually have increased levels of sodium because of added salt.

Sodium helps with the following :

- Regulate muscle contraction and nerve function
- Balance amount of fluid that the body retains or eliminates
- Regulate blood volume and blood pressure
- Regulate the acid-base balance of the blood

Why Kidney Patients Need to Monitor their Sodium Intake

Too much sodium is dangerous in people with kidney disease. The kidney, once damaged, will not be able to eliminate fluid and sodium from the body adequately, and this will cause fluid and sodium to build up in the bloodstream and tissues. When this happens, it can cause:

- Edema: swelling in the hands, legs, and face
- Increased thirst
- Shortness of breath: when fluid builds up in the lungs, it makes it difficult for one to breathe
- Heart failure: having excess fluid in the blood can make the heart to overwork itself, thereby causing it to be weak and enlarged.
- High blood pressure

How can You Monitor Your Sodium Intake

For people with kidney disease, the recommended sodium intake per day should be less than 2,000 mg. The tips below will help you to monitor your sodium intake:

- Reduce your total intake of sodium to 150 mg per snack and 400 mg per meal

- Always read food labels to check for sodium content.
- Avoid processed foods
- Pay particular attention to serving sizes.
- Cook at home without adding salt
- Compare similar brands and go for the one with the lowest sodium content.
- Go for fresh meat rather than packaged meats
- When buying spices, choose the ones that do not have salt listed in their title. For example, rather than picking garlic salt, you can pick garlic powder
- Go for fresh vegetables and fruits or no-salt-added frozen and canned produce.

Potassium

Potassium is a natural mineral found in the human body and in the foods that we eat. Potassium helps to keep the heartbeat regular and make the muscles work correctly. Potassium also helps to maintain electrolyte and fluid balance in the bloodstream. One of the functions of the kidney is to retain the right amount of potassium in the body while expelling the excess into the urine. **The** recommended potassium intake is less than 2,000 mg per day.

Why You Should Monitor Your Potassium Intake

If the kidney is damaged, it will no longer be able to discard the excess potassium, and this will cause a build-up of potassium in the body. People with kidney disease need to reduce their potassium intake to avoid blood levels from going dangerously high.

When the potassium in the blood is high, it is called hyperkalemia, and this condition can cause:

- Irregular heartbeat
- Muscle weakness
- Death
- Heart attacks
- Slow pulse

How Can You Monitor Your Intake Of Potassium?

- Keep a food journal
- Pay particular attention to serving size
- Read food labels and avoid potassium chloride
- Go for fresh vegetables and fruits
- Reduce your consumption of foods rich in potassium
- Talk with a renal dietitian to create an eating plan

- Avoid salt seasonings and substitutes with potassium
- Limit your intake of milk and dairy products to 8 ounces daily

Phosphorus

The body needs phosphorus for bone maintenance and development. The mineral also helps to develop connective organs and tissues as well as helps with muscle movement. When we consume and digest foods that contain phosphorus, the small intestines absorb the phosphorus in the food and stores it in the bones.

Why You Should Monitor Your Intake Of Phosphorus

When the kidney is active, it removes the excess phosphorus in the blood, but once the kidney is damaged, the organ will no longer be able to remove excess phosphorus which will cause the levels of phosphorus in the body to go up, and this can pull calcium from your bones thereby weakening the bones. This can also lead to dangerous deposits of calcium in the lungs, blood vessels, heart, and eyes. So, the advised dietary phosphorus is between 800 to 1,000 mg per day for most patients.

Tips on monitoring your phosphorus intake

Several foods contain phosphorus, and you need to work with your dietitian to help manage phosphorus levels. Foods high in phosphorus include:

- Milk
- Canned fish
- Cola
- Seeds
- Cheese
- Fast food
- Meat

The tips below will help you keep phosphorus at safe levels:

- Pay particular attention to serving size
- Know the foods that have low phosphorus contents
- Eat fresh vegetables and fruits
- Keep a food journal
- Confirm from your physician about the use of phosphate binders during meal

- Eat a reduced portion of foods that have high protein during meals and for snacks
- Do not go for packaged foods that have added phosphorus in them. Look out for words with "PHO" on the food label.

Protein

Protein is not harmful to a healthy kidney. When we eat foods that contain protein, it gets ingested and creates waste which the nephron of the kidney filters out. Then the additional renal proteins help to turn the waste into urine. But if the kidney is damaged, the organ will not be able to remove protein waste, and then it builds up in the blood. The recommended consumption of protein for people with chronic kidney disease differs from person to person depending on the stage of the disease. The human body needs protein for tissue maintenance and other critical bodily functions, which is why one needs to eat the rerecommended amount specific to the stage of the disease as directed by the renal dietitian or nephrologist. However, people with end-stage renal disease and undergoing dialysis have a greater need for protein.

Fluids

Patients that are in the later stages of chronic kidney disease need fluid control because excess fluid at this stage of the disease can cause a build-up of fluid in the body, which is quite dangerous. Persons undergoing dialysis have reduced urine output, and if there is an increase in the level of fluid in the body, it can put undue pressure on the patient's lungs and heart.

The allowed level of fluid per patient is calculated on an individual basis, depending on the dialysis settings and the urine output. You need to follow the fluid intake guideline as provided by your nutritionist or nephrologist To control your fluid intake for people with chronic kidney disease, you should:

- Know the amount of fluid used in cooking
- Count all the foods that can melt at room temperature like popsicles, etc.
- Do not drink more than your doctor advised you

Shopping Tips for Renal Diet

Shopping for a renal diet may seem daunting. These tips will help make things easy for you:

- Always go for fresh food

- Ensure to read the nutrition label

- Cook your meals from scratch

- When shopping, stick to the outer part of the grocery stores, where they have fresh and unboxed items.

- Plan your meals and shopping lists ahead of time

- If you have to buy canned or boxed foods, always go for those with less than 150 mg of sodium per serving.

Nutrition Label Facts

People diagnosed with kidney disease need to always monitor the amount of any substance that goes into the body. The primary way you can achieve this is by reading the nutrition labels. This means that you need to understand how to read and review these labels.

The Basics:

- **Serving size**

At the uppermost part of the nutrition label, you will find the recommended amount of food to consume at once, as well as the number of servings in one package. The service size will help with portion control. When you eat one serving of the food, it means that you also consumed all the nutrients listed on the label, and these include calories. If you consume more than one serving of a particular food, you have increased the number of nutrients consumed, the same applies when you consume less than one serving; the amount of nutrient consumed reduces.

- **Percent Daily Value (%DVs)**

These are the main regulators for nutrients like potassium, sodium, and phosphorus. When monitoring these, you need to bear in mind two basic facts about percent daily values: any substance that is 20% and above, has a high content in that serving while the substance with 5% and below %DVs has a low content.

The figure under the Percent Daily Values is for the complete 24 hours and not just for one meal or snack. What this means is that you have to add the %DVs from every source of food that you eat throughout the day to be able to calculate the exact amount of one substance you consumed for the day. You should discuss with your dietitian or nutritionist to know the foods that are safe to eat and the percent daily values number you should look for on a nutrition label.

- **Fat**

When you see total fat, know that it is a combination of saturated and unsaturated fats, monounsaturated fat, and trans fat. The primary two types of fat you need to avoid are trans fat and saturated fat because they contain chemical structures that the body cannot easily break down.

- **Protein and Carbohydrates**

If your doctor advised you to limit your intake of protein, you could still get calories from eating carbs. Carbs have three major categories, and they are fiber, starches, and sugar. Healthy sources of protein are yogurt, low-fat milk, cheese, eggs, poultry, lean meat, and beans. Before you make any dietary changes, you need to discuss it with your dietitian/ nutritionist.

- **Ingredients**

By law, food manufacturers are expected to list on the food label, all the ingredients that go into making that packaged food. The ingredients are usually written in decreasing order based on their weight. This means that the last ingredient on the list has the lowest volume in the food, while the first ingredient is the highest used in the meal.

Nutrition Facts	
Serving Size 1 cup (8 fl oz) 240 mL.	
Servings Per Container 4	
Amount Per Serving	
Calories 10 Calories from Fat 0	
	% Daily Value*
Total Fat 0g	**0**%
Saturated Fat 0g	**0**%
Trans Fat 0g	
Cholesterol 0mg	**0**%
Sodium 70mg	**3**%
Total Carbohydrate 1g	**0**%
Dietary Fiber 0g	**0**%
Sugars 0g	
Protein 2g	
Vitamin A 0% • Vitamin C 0%	
Calcium 0% • Iron 2%	
*Percent Daily Values are based on a 2,000 calorie diet.	

Foods to Avoid on Renal Diet

If the kidney gets damaged, it then becomes unable to function properly, thereby allowing waste to accumulate in the blood and fluid to build up in the body.

The good news is that limiting or avoiding certain foods in your diet can help to reduce the accumulated waste products in the blood, improve kidney function, and also prevent any further harm to the kidney. Below is a list of foods you need to avoid when following the renal diet:

Dark-coloured colas

Colas do not only give sugar and calories to the body, but they also contain additives that have phosphorus in them, particularly the dark-coloured colas. Several food manufacturers include phosphorus when processing beverages and foods to prolong shelf life, enhance flavour, and prevent discolouration. This phosphorus that the manufacturers add is much more absorbable in the human body than the natural phosphorus gotten from plants and animals.

This additive phosphorus has different contents depending on the type of cola, but it is believed that the dark-coloured colas contain about 50 to 100 mg in a 200-ml serving. It is on this basis that colas, especially the dark-coloured ones, are avoided on a renal diet.

Avocados

Avocado is known to have several nutritious values to the body, including its heart-healthy fiber, fats, and antioxidants. There is no argument that avocados are a healthy addition to one's diet, but persons with kidney disease need to avoid them because of the high content of potassium in avocados. One cup of avocado gives a massive amount of 727 mg of potassium. This is two times the amount of potassium gotten from a medium banana. For this result, you should avoid avocados, including guacamole, especially if the doctor asked you to watch your intake of potassium.

Canned Foods

We often purchase canned foods like beans, vegetables, and soups because they are more convenient and cheaper. However, a majority of these canned foods have a high amount of sodium as the food manufacturers add salt to them as a form of preservative to increase the shelf life of the product.

People with kidney disease need to limit or totally avoid canned foods because of the high amount of sodium in them. Your best choice will be to go for those labelled as "no salt added" or the low-sodium varieties.

Another helpful tip will be to drain and rinse canned foods like canned tuna and beans to reduce the amount of sodium by 33 to 80% depending on the product.

Whole Wheat Bread

It can be quite tricky for people with kidney disease to know the right bread for them. In most cases, healthy individuals are advised to go for whole wheat bread instead of refined, white flour bread because of the high fiber content in whole wheat bread. But for people with kidney disease, white bread is mostly recommended against whole wheat bread. The reason for this is because of the presence of potassium and phosphorus in whole wheat bread. The more whole grains and bran in the bread, the higher the contents of the potassium and phosphorus.

For instance, a serving of 1-ounce whole wheat bread contains approximately 69 mg of potassium and 57 mg of phosphorus. For the same serving size, white bread contains just 28 mg for both potassium and phosphorus.

Bear in mind that most bread and bread products, whether whole wheat or white bread, have high amounts of sodium. The best step is always to read the nutrition labels and compare them with the different types of bread, then choose the one that has a lower amount of sodium, if possible, while watching your portion sizes.

Brown Rice

Similar to whole wheat bread, brown rice is a whole grain that is rich in phosphorus and potassium, more than the white rice. One cup of cooked brown rice contains 154 mg of potassium and 150 mg of phosphorus, while one cup of cooked white rice contains only 54 mg of potassium and 69 mg of phosphorus.

You do not need to remove brown rice from your diet totally, but you need to have a controlled portion while balancing it with other foods to avoid excess daily intake of phosphorus and potassium. Other lower phosphorus and nutritious grains that you can substitute for brown rice are couscouses, pearled barley, buckwheat and bulgur.

Bananas

Bananas have a very high potassium content but naturally low in sodium. A medium banana gives approximately 422 mg of potassium. It may be challenging to maintain a daily potassium intake of 2,000 mg if you consume banana daily. Unfortunately, several other tropical fruits also have high potassium contents. But pineapples contain lesser potassium contents than other tropical fruits, and you can take pineapples in place of bananas.

Dairy

Dairy products have a rich amount of several nutrients and vitamins. They are also natural sources of potassium and phosphorus, as well as protein. For instance, 1 cup of whole milk gives approximately 349 mg of potassium and 222 mg of phosphorus.

Yet, it could be dangerous for persons with kidney disease to consume too much dairy added with other foods rich in phosphorus as it can cause damage to bone health. This may come as a surprise to you mainly because we all know that dairy and milk are good for muscle health and healthy bones. But, if the kidneys are damaged, consuming too much phosphorus can cause the mineral to buildup in the blood. Once this happens, the bones become weak and thin over time, thereby increasing your risk of bone fracture or breakage.

Dairy products are also rich in protein. One cup of whole milk gives about 8 grams of protein. People with kidney disease should reduce their intake of dairy to avoid protein waste building up in the blood.

Almond milk and enriched rice milk have lower contents of protein, phosphorus, and potassium than cow's milk, and they are better alternatives for people following the renal diet.

Oranges and Orange Juice

Oranges and orange juice are rich in Vitamin C as well as potassium. One large orange gives approximately 333 mg of potassium. While one cup of orange juice has about 473 mg of potassium. Because of the high content of potassium, people on a renal diet need to limit or totally avoid oranges and orange juice.

For people following the renal diets, you can replace oranges and orange juice with cranberries, apples, and grapes along with their respective juices.

Processed Meat

Over the years, processed meat has been associated with chronic diseases and considered unhealthy because of the presence of preservatives. Processed meats are meats that have been dried, salted, canned, or cured. These include sausage, pepperoni, jerky, bacon, and hot dogs. Typically, processed meat has a large amount of salts used to preserve flavor and improve the taste. If you eat a lot of processed meat, you may find it hard to maintain a daily sodium intake level of less than 2,000 mg.

Also, processed meat has high protein content. If your doctor has asked that you watch your protein intake, then you have another reason to reduce your consumption of processed meat.

Olives, Pickles, and Relish
Relish, processed olives, and pickles are all examples of pickled or cured foods. Usually, during the pickling or curing process, a lot of salt is added to complete the process. For instance, one pickle spear has a sodium content of over 300 mg. In the same vein, you will find 244 mg of sodium in 2 tablespoons of sweet pickle relish.

Processed olives are not left out as they are saltier because they are fermented and cured to reduce the bitter taste. Five green pickled olives give about 195 mg of sodium, which is very high for a small serving. Several grocery stores carry reduced-sodium options of relish, olives, and pickles, which have less sodium than the traditional versions.

However, these reduced-sodium options may also have high sodium content, so it is safer to watch your consumption of these foods.

Apricots

Apricots are rich sources of Vitamin A, vitamin C, and fiber. Let's not forget that they are also rich in potassium. For example, one cup of fresh apricots gives approximately 427 mg of potassium. Also, dried apricots have more concentrated potassium content: one cup of dried apricots gives about 1,500 mg of potassium. This means that one cup of dried apricot will provide you with 75 percent of the 2,000 mg low-potassium advised for people on a renal diet. For this reason, it is advisable to remove apricots, especially dried apricots, from your diet when on a renal diet.

Potatoes and Sweet Potatoes

These foods have a high potassium content. For example, one medium-sized baked potato gives about 610 mg of potassium, while one average-sized baked sweet potato gives about 541 mg of potassium.

The good news is that you can soak or bleach some high-potassium foods like potatoes and sweet potatoes, to reduce their potassium contents.

To reduce the potassium content by approximately 50%, cut the potatoes into small, thin pieces, and boil them for a minimum of 10 minutes. Research has proven that when you soak potatoes in a large pot of water for a minimum of 4 hours before cooking, you have succeeded in reducing the amount of potassium in the potatoes than the ones that were not soaked before cooking. This method is also called the 'double cook method' or 'potassium leaching.'

Note that this method does not totally remove the potassium in the food; it only reduces the potassium content of the potatoes. A considerable amount of potassium will still be found in the potatoes, so you still need to practice portion control to maintain the amount of potassium that you consume.

Tomatoes

This is another fruit that has high potassium content and may not be suitable for the renal diet. Tomatoes can be stewed or served raw and are sometimes used to make sauces. One cup of tomato sauce can provide a minimum of 900 mg of potassium. Unfortunately for persons following the renal diet, tomatoes are present in several dishes. But, you can substitute tomatoes with foods like roasted red pepper sauce and still get that delicious taste while reducing the potassium content.

Pre-made, Packaged And Instant Meals

Processed foods are one major source of sodium in a diet. When compared to other foods, pre-made, packaged, and instant meals are the most heavily processed, and for this reason, they contain the highest amount of sodium. Examples include instant noodles, microwavable meals, and pizza. It will be challenging to maintain the daily 2,000 mg intake of sodium if most of your meals include these highly processed foods. Not only do these heavily processed foods have a high volume of sodium in them, but they also do not give any nutrients to the body.

Beet Greens, Spinach and Swiss Chard

Beet greens, spinach, and Swiss Chard are leafy greens that are rich in several minerals and nutrients, including potassium. When you serve these vegetables raw, they contain about 140 to 290 mg of potassium per cup.

Although these leafy greens shrink to a smaller size when cooked, it doesn't reduce the potassium content. For example, when you cook half-cup of raw spinach, it shrinks to about one tablespoon while maintaining the same amount of potassium content. So, consuming half-cup of cooked spinach means that you are consuming more potassium than when you eat half-cup of raw spinach.

The best way to avoid excess consumption of potassium is by eating a moderate serving of beet greens, spinach, and Swiss Chards in their raw form as against the cooked greens.

Prunes, Raisins, and Dates

Prunes, raisins, and dates are common dried fruits. When fruits are dried, all the nutrients in them become concentrated, and this includes potassium. For instance, four Dates give approximately 688 mg of potassium, while one cup of prunes provides about 1,274 mg of potassium, which is about five times the amount of potassium found in one cup of plums.

Because these fruits have high potassium contents, people on the renal diet need to avoid consuming these fruits if they want to maintain the advised potassium levels.

Crackers, Chips, and Pretzels

Snacks that are ready to eat like crackers, chips, and Pretzels not only lack nutrients but also have high salt content. It is also easy for one to eat more than the advised portion sizes for these foods, and the more you consume these foods, the more salts you consume. Let's not forget that eating chips made from potatoes will increase the amount of potassium in the body.

Best Foods to Eat with Kidney Disease

We have talked about the foods that you should limit or avoid when following the renal diet. Again, I need to remind you that every person with kidney disease differs from the next person, and so, you need to talk with your health care provider about your specific dietary needs. While we have seen a long list of foods to limit or avoid, the good news is that several healthy and delicious meals are low in sodium, potassium, and phosphorus.

Below are 20 of the best foods that people with kidney diseases can eat.

Cauliflower

This is a nutritious vegetable rich in several nutrients like B vitamin folate, vitamins K and vitamin C. It is also a rich source of anti-inflammatory compounds like indoles. Cauliflower is also an excellent source of fiber. If you are looking for a low potassium side dish that can replace potatoes, you should try mashed cauliflower.

One cup of cooked cauliflower contains the following:

- Phosphorus: 40 mg

- Potassium: 176 mg

- Sodium: 19 mg

Blueberries

Blueberries are one of the best sources of antioxidants and are packed with nutrients. These berries are sweet and contain antioxidants known as anthocyanins, which help to protect us from certain cancers, heart disease, diabetes, and cognitive decline. They are an excellent choice for the renal diet as they are low in potassium, phosphorus, and sodium.

One cup of fresh blueberries contains the following:

- Phosphorus: 18 mg

- Potassium: 114 mg

- Sodium: 1.5 mg

Sea bass

This food is rich in quality protein and contains healthy fats called omega-3s. These omega-3s helps to reduce inflammation as well as reduce the risk of anxiety, depression, and cognitive decline. Although all fish have high phosphorus contents, sea bass is known to have a lower amount of phosphorus than other seafood. Still, you should consume this food in small portions to maintain your phosphorus levels at the advised level.

85 grams/ 3-ounces of cooked sea bass contains the following:

- Phosphorus: 211 mg

- Potassium: 279 mg

- Sodium: 74 mg

Red grapes

These fruits are not just delicious but also rich in nutrition. They are rich in vitamin C and contain antioxidants known as flavonoids, which helps to reduce inflammation.

Also, red grapes have a high content of resveratrol, a type of flavonoids that is beneficial to heart health as well as protect the body against cognitive decline and diabetes. They are an excellent addition to the kidney-friendly diet.

75 grams/ half cup of red grapes contain the following:

- Phosphorus: 15 mg
- Potassium: 144 mg
- Sodium: 1.5 mg

Egg Whites

Egg yolks are very nutritious, but they have high phosphorus contents. For persons following the renal diet, the egg whites are more beneficial as they give a high-quality and kidney-friendly type of protein.

Also, egg whites are excellent for people undergoing dialysis, who needs to increase their protein intake while limiting the amount of phosphorus they consume.

66 grams or two large egg whites will give you the following

- Phosphorus: 10 mg
- Potassium: 108 mg
- Sodium: 110 mg

Garlic

People that have kidney problems need to limit their sodium intake, and this includes added salt. You can use garlic in place of salt to add flavor to your dish while providing other nutritional benefits. Garlic is rich in Vitamin C and B6, manganese as well as sulfur compounds that contain anti-inflammatory properties.

9 grams/ three cloves of garlic contain the following:

- Phosphorus: 14 mg
- Potassium: 36 mg
- Sodium: 1.5 mg

Buckwheat

Several whole grains have high phosphorus content, but buckwheat is one healthy exception. This food is highly nutritious and rich in fibers, iron, magnesium, and B vitamins. It is also a gluten-free grain, which makes it a good choice for people with gluten intolerance or celiac disease. In my celiac diet book, I talked extensively on how to follow and succeed with the celiac diet for persons with celiac disease or glucose intolerance.

84 grams/ half cup of cooked buckwheat contains the following

- Phosphorus: 59 mg

- Potassium: 74 mg

- Sodium: 3.5 mg

Olive Oil

Olive oil is a great addition for people with kidney disease as it has no phosphorous in it and contains healthy fat. In some cases, people with advanced kidney disease are not able to keep weight on, and for this, they need to eat healthy foods that contain high calories like olive oil.

Most of the fat found in olive oil is monounsaturated fat known as folic acid, which has anti-inflammatory properties. Also, another reason olive oil is a healthy choice for cooking is that these monounsaturated fats remain stable under high temperatures.

23.5 grams or one tablespoon of olive oil contains:

- Phosphorus: 0 mg

- Potassium: 0.1 mg

- Sodium: 0.3 mg

Bulgur

Bulgur is unlike other whole grains wheat products that have high potassium and phosphorus contents. This grain is nutritious and rich in manganese, iron, magnesium, and B vitamins. Bulgur is not only rich in plant-based protein but is also a rich source of dietary fiber.

91-gram/ half-cup serving of bulgur contains the following:

- Phosphorus: 36 mg
- Potassium: 62 mg
- Sodium: 4.5 mg

Cabbage

This vegetable, which belongs to the cruciferous vegetable family, is rich in minerals, vitamins, and powerful plant compounds. It is also rich in Vitamin C, vitamin K as well as several B vitamins. Cabbage also provides insoluble fiber; this is a type of fiber that helps to promote a healthy digestive system by encouraging regular bowel movements and adding bulk to stool. The good news is that this vegetable has a low content of sodium, phosphorus, and potassium.

70 grams/ one cup of shredded cabbage contains the following:

- Phosphorus: 18 mg
- Potassium: 119 mg
- Sodium: 13 mg

Skinless Chicken

While some people with kidney disease need to limit their protein intake, the body needs high-quality protein to stay healthy. Chicken breast without the skin has less sodium, potassium, and phosphorus than the ones with skin on. When shopping, always go for fresh chickens and avoid pre-made roasted chicken as they have high amounts of phosphorus and sodium.

84 grams or three ounces of skinless chicken breast gives:

- Phosphorus: 192 mg
- Potassium: 216 mg
- Sodium: 63 mg

Bell Peppers

Bell peppers are low in potassium and nutrients. These peppers contain powerful antioxidants vitamin C. One small red bell pepper is enough to provide 105% of the recommended vitamin C intake. This vegetable is also rich in Vitamin A, a vital nutrient for immune function, which is often missing in people with kidney disease.

74 grams/ one small red pepper provides
- Phosphorus: 19 mg
- Potassium: 156 mg
- Sodium: 3 mg

Onions

Onion is a great source of sodium-free flavors to add to your renal diet meals. It may be challenging for several people to reduce their salt intake because of the flavor that salt adds to the meal, and the only way to eliminate salt from our meals is to find a flavorful alternative. If you need to add flavor to your meals without it having any negative effects on your kidney, you can saute onions with olive oil and garlic.

Also, onions are rich in B vitamins, manganese, vitamin C, and prebiotic fibers that help the digestive system to stay healthy by feeding it with beneficial gut bacteria.

70 grams/ one small onion provides the following:

- Phosphorus: 20 mg
- Potassium: 102 mg
- Sodium: 3 mg

Arugula

Several healthy greens like kale and spinach have high contents of potassium and are not fit for the renal diet. But, Arugula has low potassium content, which makes it a great choice for renal diet side dishes, and salads. Arugula is rich in vitamin K, calcium, and manganese, which are all important minerals and nutrients for bone health. This vegetable also contains nitrates that help to lower blood pressure, an added advantage for those with kidney disease.

A 20-gram/ one cup of raw arugula contains:

- Phosphorus: 10 mg
- Potassium: 74 mg
- Sodium: 6 mg

Macadamia nuts

Most of the nuts available are not for people on a renal diet because of the high phosphorus contents. But the macadamia nuts are a delicious exception for people with kidney problems. They have low phosphorus contents, unlike popular nuts like almonds and peanuts. They are also rich in B vitamins, healthy fats, manganese, magnesium, iron, and copper.

28 grams or one ounce of macadamia nit provides the following:

- Phosphorus: 53 mg
- Potassium: 103 mg

- Sodium: 1.4 mg

Radish

These are crunchy veggies that make healthy additions to the kidney-friendly diet. They are very low in phosphorus and potassium but high in several other important nutrients. Radishes are rich in vitamin C, a helpful antioxidant proven to reduce the risk of cataracts and heart disease. The peppery taste of this vegetable can serve as flavor to low sodium dishes.

58 grams/ half cup of sliced radishes provides:

- Phosphorus: 12 mg
- Potassium: 135 mg
- Sodium: 23 mg

Turnips

You can use Turnips to replace other vegetables that have high potassium content like winter squash and potatoes. This vegetable comes loaded with vitamin c and fiber. They also have a good amount of manganese and vitamin B6. You can boil/ roast and mash them for a healthy side dish for persons on a renal diet.

78 grams or a half cup of cooked turnips provides the following:

- Phosphorus: 20 mg
- Potassium: 138 mg
- Sodium: 12.5 mg

Pineapples

Several tropical fruits like kiwis, bananas, and oranges have high potassium contents. The good news is, pineapple with its low potassium content, is a sweet alternative for these tropical fruits for people with kidney disease. Pineapple is rich in vitamin C, manganese, fiber, and bromelain, an enzyme that helps to fight inflammation.

165 grams or 1 cup of pineapple chunks provides:

- Phosphorus: 13 mg
- Potassium: 180 mg
- Sodium: 2 mg

Cranberries

This fruit is both beneficial to the kidneys and the urinary tract. It contains phytonutrients known as A-type proanthocyanidins that stop bacteria from sticking to the lining of the bladder and the urinary tract, ultimately, preventing infection. Persons with kidney disease have a higher risk of urinary tract infections; however, taking this fruit will reduce your chances of getting infections. You can enjoy cranberries fresh, cooked, dried, or in its juice form. Also, cranberries have low contents of sodium, phosphorus, and potassium.

100 grams/ one cup of fresh cranberries provides:

- Phosphorus: 11 mg
- Potassium: 80 mg
- Sodium: 2 mg

Shiitake Mushrooms

This food is your best bet if you are following the renal diet and need a plant-based food to substitute meat and also reduce your intake of protein. These savory ingredients are excellent sources of copper, selenium, manganese, and vitamins. They also provide a rich amount of dietary fiber and plant-based protein.

Shiitake mushrooms are a better choice for people on a renal diet than white button mushrooms and portobello because of its low potassium content

145 grams/ one cup of cooked shiitake mushrooms provide the following:

- Phosphorus: 42 mg

- Potassium: 170 mg

- Sodium 6 mg

Portion Control

When you choose to eat healthy meals, you have taken the first step to total healing; however, overeating of even healthy foods can cause problems for the body. We have established the importance of eating a healthy diet, and the next step is to know how much of these healthy foods to eat. This is what is referred to as **Portion Control**

The tips below will help you control the portions of foods that you eat:

- The nutrition facts label on food will tell you the serving size and the amount of each available nutrient in one serving. Several packages have more than one serving. For instance, the serving size of a 20-ounce bottle of soda is actually two and a half sizes. Several fresh foods like vegetables and fruits do not have any nutrition facts labels. You should meet with your dietitian to provide you with a list of nutrition facts for fresh foods and the ways to measure the right portions.

- Do not rush the food; take your time to chew slowly, and once you are no more hungry, ensure to stop eating. It takes approximately 20 minutes for the stomach to signal the brain that you are full. If you rush your food, you may end up eating more than you need.
- As much as possible, do not eat while occupied with something else like driving or watching TV. Distractions may cause you to eat more than you should without realizing it.
- Do not eat directly from the food package, but instead, take out your desired serving and keep the box or bag away.

Generally, it is critical to practice portion control when planning your meals. This is more emphasized when following the renal diet due to the restriction or reduction of intake of certain foods and drinks.

CHAPTER 2: BREAKFAST RECIPES

40 – Second Omelet

Prep time – 5 mins

Cook time – 5 mins

Total time – 10 mins

Ingredients:

(1 serving)

- Two eggs
- One tablespoon of unsalted butter
- Two tablespoons of water
- ½ cup of filling either seafood, vegetables, or fruits

Instruction:

- Beat the eggs and water until they are thoroughly blended.
- Heat the butter in a 10-inch fry pan until it's hot enough to sizzle a drop of water.
- Pour the egg mixture into the pan and allow the mixture to spread to the edges of the pan. Use an inverted pancake flipper to push the cooked part of the egg to the middle, allowing the uncooked portion to spread to the hot fry pan surface. You

could also tilt the pan, if necessary. Do this until the egg is set and ceases to flow.

- Fill the omelet with ½ cup of whatever filling you like; fruit, meat, vegetable, or seafood. If you're right-handed, put the filling on the left side, and if you are left-handed, put the filling on the right side.

- Use the pancake flipper to fold the omelet into two halves, then turn it into a plate with the bottom facing upwards.

- Serve!

Nutritional facts:

for one serving per recipe

Calories   255

Carbohydrates. 1.3 g

Dietary fiber   2 g

Phosphorus   195mg

Potassium   122 mg

Protein   13 g

Sodium   145 mg

60 – Seconds Salsa

Prep time – 1 min

Cook time – 1 min

Total time – 2 min

Ingredients:

(8 servings)

- green onions - 2 (chopped)
- plum or Roma tomatoes, chopped - 4
- green bell pepper – ½ (chopped)
- minced garlic (3 cloves)
- fresh cilantro- ½ bunch (chopped)
- fresh jalapeño – ½ (chopped)
- cumin - ½ teaspoon
- fresh oregano – ¼ (chopped) or dried oregano- 1 tablespoon

Instruction:

- Mix all the ingredients using a blender or a food processor, until the larger ingredients become small and chunky.
- Allow to sit in the freezer for a few hours
- Serve once chilled with plain tortilla chips

Nutritional facts:

Calories   14

Carbohydrates   2 g

Dietary fiber   0 g

Phosphorus   14 mg

Potassium   117 mg

Protein   1 g

Sodium   4 mg

Fat   1 g

Baked acorn squash with pineapple

Prep time – 15 min

Cook time – 45 min

Total time – 1 hour

Ingredients:

(2 servings)

- Pineapple - 3 tablespoons (crushed)
- Acorn squash – 1 (cut in half and seeded)
- Brown sugar (2 teaspoons)
- Unsalted butter (1 tablespoon + 2 teaspoons)
- Nutmeg - ¼ teaspoon

Instruction:

- Preheat your oven to 400 degrees

- Place the squash in a greased baking pan, with the cut side facing up
- Add a teaspoon of brown sugar and a teaspoon of butter to each half of the squash
- Cover the squash with an aluminum foil and bake for approximately 30 minutes or until tender
- Scoop the cooked squash out of the shell, leaving about ¼ inch thick shell
- Mix the pineapple, cooked squash, nutmeg, and one tablespoon of butter. Beat until the mixture gets smooth
- Scoop the mixture back into the shells and bake for about 15 minutes, at 425 degrees.

Nutritional facts:

Calories   202

Carbohydrates   31 g

Phosphorus   80 mg

Potassium   783 mg

Protein   2 g

Sodium   90 mg

Anytime Energy Bars

Prep time – 10 min

Cook time – 40 min

Total time – 50 min

Ingredients:

(8 servings)

- Rolled oats (1 cup)
- Unsalted peanuts – 3 tablespoons (chopped)
- Ground cinnamon (½ teaspoon)
- Semi-sweet mini chocolate chips (1/4 cup)
- Shredded coconuts (1/3 cup)
- Honey (3 tablespoons)
- Applesauce (1/3 cup)
- Eggs – 3 large

Instruction:

- Heat up your oven to 325 degrees.
- Apply cooking spray on a 9-by-9-inch pan.
- Add the cinnamon, oats, coconut, peanuts, and chocolate chips to a large mixing bowl.
- In another bowl, beat the eggs then add honey and applesauce. Mix very well.

- Add the oat mixture with the egg mixture. Mix thoroughly.
- Evenly spread the mixture into the bottom of the already greased pan.
- Cook for approximately 40 minutes. Allow to cool before you cut into square bars.
- You may place it in an airtight container and keep refrigerated for up to a week.

Nutritional facts:

Calories 206

Carbohydrates   27 g

Dietary fibers   8 g

Phosphorus

Potassium

Protein 7 g

Sodium   35 mg

Apple Filled Crepes

Prep time – 5 min

Cook time – 20 seconds

Total time – 5 min 20 seconds

Ingredients:

(1 serving)

- Egg yolks (4)
- Whole eggs (2)
- Sugar (½ a cup)
- Flour (a cup)
- Oil (¼ cup)
- Milk(2 cups)
- Apples (4)
- Brown sugar (½ a cup)
- Cinnamon (½ a teaspoon)
- Nutmeg (½ teaspoon)
- Unsalted butter (1/2 cup or one stick)

Instruction:

- Put the whole eggs, egg yolks, oil, flour, sugar, and milk into a bowl and mix until there are no lumps in the mixture.
- On medium heat, heat a small-sized non-stick skillet pan.
- Spray the pan with cooking spray.

- Use ¼ cup or 2-ounce ladle to spoon a scoop of the crepe batter into the pan, then tilt the frypan to allow the batter spread thinly on the frypan.
- Cook for approximately 20 seconds before you turn the crepe to the other side using a rubber spatula then cook for another ten more seconds.
- Set the crepes aside and prepare the filling.
- Peel all the apples, then core and cut them into 12 slices.
- Heat a medium-sized sauté pan.
- Melt the butter in the pan and add the brown sugar once hot.
- Add the cinnamon, apples, and nutmeg to the sauté pan and cook until the apples are tender but not mushy. Set the pan aside and allow it to cool.
- Assemble the crepes by filling the middle of each crepe with approximately two tablespoons of the Apple filling.
- Then roll the crepe into a log.

Note: You can make this meal well ahead of consumption time, just use a plastic wrap to cover and place in the refrigerator. Whenever you want to eat, put in the microwave for a few seconds.

Nutritional facts:

Calories   315

Carbohydrates   40 g

Dietary fibers   15 g

Phosphorus   103 mg

Potassium 160 mg

Protein   5 g

Sodium   356 mg

Banana Oat Smoothie

Prep time – 2 min

Cook time – 30 seconds

Total time – 2 min 30 seconds

Ingredients:

(2 servings)

- Chilled cooked oatmeal (½ a cup)
- Skimmed milk (2/3 of a cup)
- Brown sugar (2 tablespoons)
- Wheat germ (1 tablespoon)

- Vanilla extract (1 ½ teaspoon)
- ½ frozen bananas – dice into chunks

Instruction:

- Put the oatmeal in a blender and puree for a few minutes.
- Add the banana, the milk, the wheat germ, brown sugar, and vanilla. Blend the mixture until it is thick and smooth.

Nutritional facts:

Calories   172

Carbohydrates   33 g

Phosphorus   160 mg

Potassium   297 mg

Protein   6 g

Sodium   42 mg

Berry smoothie

Prep time – 30 seconds

Cook time – 30 seconds

Total time – 60 seconds

Ingredients:

(2 servings)

- Cranberry juice cocktail (¼ cup)
- Firm silken tofu (2/3 cup)
- Frozen unsweetened blueberries, (½ cup)
- Frozen unsweetened raspberries, (½ cup)
- Vanilla extract (1 teaspoon)
- Powdered lemonade (½teaspoon)

Instruction:

- Pour the cranberry juice in a blender.
- Add the tofu, raspberries, blueberries, vanilla extract, and lemonade powder.
- Blend until the mixture is very smooth.
- Serve immediately and enjoy!

Nutritional facts:

Calories   115

Carbohydrates   18 g

Dietary fibers.   1 g

Phosphorus.   80 mg

Potassium.   233 mg

Protein.   6 g

Sodium.   14 mg

Fat   3 g

Blueberry square bars

Prep time – 30 minutes

Cook time – 1 hour

Total time – 1 hour 30 minutes

Ingredients:

(16 servings)

- 3 cups of blueberries
- 1 ½ cups of flour
- One teaspoon of cinnamon
- A cup of oats
- A cup of sugar
- 1 ½ sticks or ¾ cup of melted butter (preferably unsalted)
- zest of 1 lemon
- ¾ cup of sugar
- Three tablespoons of cornstarch
- A cup of water

Instruction:

- Preheat your oven to 350 degrees.

- In a medium-sized bowl, mix the oats, flour, sugar, cinnamon, and butter until the mixture is crumbly.
- Put ½ of the oat and flour mixture into a 9-inch square pan.
- Throw in the blueberries with the lemon zest and cover the bottom of the pan.
- Mix the sugar and corn starch in a microwaveable bowl, slowly stir in water, and put to heat just until it begins to boil.
- Pour the sugar, cornstarch and water mixture over the blueberries.
- Pour the remaining oat and flour mixture over the top.
- Cook for approximately 45 minutes to 1 hour
- Serve!

Nutritional facts:

For 16 servings per recipe

Calories.   247

Carbohydrates. 40 g

Phosphorus.   17 mg

Potassium.   38 mg

Protein.   2g

Sodium.   3 mg

Spicy Tofu Scramble

Prep time – 5 min

Cook time – 20 min

Total time – 25 min

Ingredients:

(2 servings)

- Olive oil - 1 teaspoon

- Green bell pepper - ¼ cup (chopped)

- Red bell pepper - ¼ cup (chopped)

- Firm tofu- 1 cup (go for the one that is less than 10% calcium)

- Garlic powder - ¼ teaspoon

- Onion powder - 1 teaspoon

- Turmeric - ⅛ teaspoon

- Garlic - 1 clove (minced)

Instruction:

- Sauté the green bell pepper, red bell pepper, and garlic in olive oil using a medium non-stick skillet pan.

- Rinse, drain the tofu, and crumble into the skillet.

- Add the other ingredients that are yet to be added.

- Stir and cook on low to medium heat for about 20 minutes or until the tofu turns light golden brown. There will be no more water in the mixture.

- Serve warm!

Nutritional facts:

Calories. 213

Carbohydrates.   10 g

Dietary fibers.   2 g

Phosphorus.   242 mg

Potassium.   467 mg

Protein.   18 g

Sodium   24 mg

Stuffed Breakfast Biscuits

Prep time – 5 min

Cook time – 15 min

Total time – 20 min

Ingredients:

(12 servings)

- sugar or honey - 1 tablespoon
- Flour - 2 cups
- baking soda - ½ teaspoon
- softened unsalted butter - 8 tablespoons
- lemon juice - 1 tablespoon
- milk - ¾ cup

For Filling:

- Reduced sodium bacon – 8 ounces (chopped)
- Eggs – 4
- scallions - ¼ cup (thinly sliced)
- Cheddar cheese- 1 cup (shredded)

Instruction:

- Preheat oven to 425 degrees
- To prepare the filling, scramble the eggs leaving it slightly undercooked.
- Cook the bacon until it becomes crispy.
- Mix all four ingredients for filling and keep aside.

To prepare the dough,

- Add all the dry ingredients into a large bowl.

- Use a pastry cutter or a fork to cut in the unsalted butter in pea sizes.

- Make a hole in the center of the dough, then knead in the lemon juice and milk.

- Place liners on the muffin tins or lightly apply oil and flour on the sides and bottoms of the muffin tins

- Scoop the mix into the muffin tins, ¼ cup of mixture per muffin tins.

- Bake at 425 degrees for approximately 12 minutes or until the dough turns golden brown.

Nutritional facts:

Calories.   330

Carbohydrates   19 g

Dietary fibers.   1 g

Phosphorus.   170 mg.

Potassium   152 mg

Protein.   11 g

Sodium   329 mg

Buttermilk Pancakes

Prep time – 5 min

Cook time – 3 min

Total time – 8 min

Ingredients:

(9 servings)

- All-purpose flour - 2 cups

- Cream of tartar - 1 teaspoon

- Baking soda - 1½ teaspoons

- Sugar - 2 tablespoons

- Low-fat buttermilk - 2 cups

- Eggs -2 large

- Canola oil - ¼ cup

- One tablespoon of canola oil for cooking

Instruction:

- Heat a pan over medium heat.

- Put the flour, baking soda, and sugar in a bowl and mix.

- Mix the buttermilk, canola oil, and egg in a separate bowl.

- Add the dry ingredients to the wet mixture.

- Grease the pan with a tablespoon of canola oil.

- Use a 1/3 measuring cup to scoop the mixture into the pan. Let the pancakes spread about 4-inches across. Ensure to leave about 2 inches between each pancake for easy flipping.

- When the bubbles at the top of each pancake are almost gone, use a spatula to flip the pancakes.
- Allow the flipped side to turn brown until the middle no longer looks wet.
- You can serve with a side of eggs and fresh berries for a healthier twist.

Nutritional facts:

Calories.   217

Carbohydrates   27g

Dietary fibers   1 g

Phosphorus.   100 mg

Potassium   182 mg

Protein   6 g

Sodium.   330 mg

Burrito

Prep time – 5 min

Cook time – 2 min 20 seconds

Total time – 7 minutes 30 seconds

Ingredients:

(2 servings)

- Eggs - 4
- green chilli - 3 tablespoons (Diced)
- Ground cumin - ¼ teaspoon
- Hot pepper sauce - ½ teaspoon
- Flour tortillas – 2 (Burrito size)
- Salsa – 2 tablespoons

Instruction:

- Place a medium-sized pan over medium heat after spraying it with non-stick cooking spray.
- Beat the eggs in a bowl and add your diced green chilies, hot sauce, and ground cumin.
- Pour the egg mixture into the pan and cook-stir for about 2 minutes, until the egg is done.
- Heat the flour tortillas in another pan over medium heat or in the microwave for about 20 seconds.
- Divide the egg mixture into two halves and place each half on each tortilla before you roll it into a burrito.

- Serve the burritos with a tablespoon of salsa each.

Nutritional facts:

Calories.   257

Carbohydrates   20 g

Dietary fibers.   2 g

Phosphorus   184 mg

Potassium   246 mg

Protein   15 g

Sodium   384 mg

Parsley Burger

Prep time – 10 min

Cook time – 15 min

Total time – 25 min

Ingredients:

(4 servings)

- Ground beef or turkey - 1 pound

- Chopped Parsley - 1 tablespoon

- Lemon juice - 1 tablespoon

- Black pepper - ¼ teaspoon

- Ground thyme - ¼ teaspoon

- Oregano - ¼ teaspoon

Instruction:

- Put the ground beef or turkey in a bowl, add the other ingredients, and mix properly.

- Shape the mixture into patties.

- Place a lightly greased pan on low heat.

- Place the patties in the pan and cook for approximately 15 minutes.

Nutritional facts:

Calories   171

Phosphorus.   180 mg

Potassium   289 mg

Protein   20 g

Sodium   108 mg

Tuna Mayonnaise Pasta

Ingredients:

(1 serving)

- pasta shells (90 g)

- A can of tuna (200 g)

- Chopped spring onions (2)

- Low-fat mayonnaise (2 tablespoons)

- canned sweetcorn (2 tablespoons)

- Diced tomatoes (1)

- Chopped coriander (a handful)

- Pepper flakes (to taste)

Instruction:

- Cook the pasta as directed on the packet.

- Drain the pasta and put it in a bowl

- Drain the tuna and the sweetcorn out of their respective cans and add them to the pasta along with the spring onions, and parsley

- Add the mayonnaise and mix until everything is completely coated

- Add pepper to taste

- Add tomato to garnish

- Serve!

Nutritional facts:

Calories   322.4

Carbohydrates.   37.2 g

Dietary fibers.   2.0 g

Potassium.   152.1 mg

Protein.   17.4 g

Sodium.   222.3 mg

Coleslaw

Prep time – 10 min

Cook time – 0 min

Total time – 10 min

Ingredients:

(10 servings)

- Coleslaw mix with cabbage and carrots - 1 pound/ 1 bag
- Mayonnaise - 1 cup
- Apple cider vinegar - 2 teaspoons
- Horseradish - 1 tablespoon
- Granulated sugar - 3 tablespoons
- Fresh dill - 2 teaspoons (chopped)

Instruction:

- Mix the mayonnaise, horseradish, sugar, vinegar, and dill in a large bowl.
- Add the coleslaw mix and stir until well blended.

- Chill for at least 1 hour. Best to chill overnight before serving.

Nutritional facts:

For ten servings per recipe

Calories   107

Carbohydrates   8 g

Potassium   117 mg

Phosphorus   11 mg

Protein   0 g

Sodium   170 mg

Quiche

Prep time – 5 min

Cook time – 60 min

Total time – 1 hour 5 min

Ingredients

(6 servings)

- Eggs (6)

- 2% milk (1 cup)

- Total filling (2 cups)

- Grated cheese (4 ounces)

- P-inch deep-dish frozen pie shell

Instruction:

- Preheat your oven to 350 degrees.

- Add the eggs, milk, cheese, and filling (leftover vegetables or meat such as chicken, onions, asparagus, or mushrooms) in a bowl and mix thoroughly. If you have a high level of phosphorous, use only two ounces of cheese.

- Pour the mixture into the frozen pie shell.

- Bake for about 50 to 60 minutes. Insert a toothpick; if it comes out clean, it means your food is ready.

- Allow to cool for about 5 minutes before you cut.

Nutritional facts:

For six servings per recipe

Calories   356

Carbohydrates   24 g

Dietary fibers.   22 g

Phosphorus.   278 mg

Potassium.   257 mg

Protein   16 g

Sodium.   409 mg

Pumpkin bread

Prep time – 10 min

Cooking time – 60 min

Total time – 1 hour 10 min

Ingredients:

(12 servings)

- Unsweetened applesauce (1 ½ cups)
- Brown sugar (1 cup)
- Vegetable oil (½ a cup)
- Eggs (2)
- All-purpose flour (2 cups)
- Baking soda (1 teaspoon)
- Baking powder (½ a teaspoon)
- Pumpkin pie spice (2 teaspoons)

Instruction:

- Preheat your oven to 350 degrees.
- Grease the loaf pan with some oil.
- Put the brown sugar, applesauce, oil, and eggs together in a medium-sized bowl and whisk properly.

- Mix the flour, baking soda, baking powder, and pumpkin pie spice in another bowl.
- Add the wet mixture to the dry mixture and stir until properly combined.
- Pour the batter into your loaf pan.
- Bake for about 50-60 minutes.
- Check if it's done by poking with a toothpick, which should come out clean.

Nutritional facts:

For 12 servings per recipe

Calories   252

Carbohydrates   38 g

Dietary fiber   10g

Phosphorus   41 mg

Potassium   82 mg

Protein   3 g

Sodium   141 mg

Rhubarb bread

Prep time – 10 min

Cook time – 40 min

Total time – 50 min

Ingredients:

(20 servings)

- Diced rhubarb (1 ½ cups)
- Vegetable oil (2/3 cup)
- Brown sugar - 1 ½ cups
- Egg – 1
- Yogurt or Sour milk (1 cup)
- Vanilla (a teaspoon)
- Baking soda (a teaspoon)
- All-purpose flour (2 ½ cups)
- Chopped nuts (1½ cup)

Instruction:

- Mix the egg, sour milk, vegetable oil, and vanilla in a bowl.
- Mix the brown sugar, flour, and baking soda in another bowl.
- Stir the wet and dry ingredients together until they're properly mixed.
- Add the chopped nuts and diced rhubarb and mix properly.

- Grease two loaf pans and dust them with flour. Pour the batter into the two pans.

- Bake for approximately 40 minutes at 325 degrees F.

- Mix 1 tablespoon of melted butter and ½ cup of sugar and drizzle over the loaves.

- Cut into slices and serve warm.

- Could be served with a sauce or dip

Nutrition Facts:

For 20 servings per recipe.

Calories	195
Potassium	117 mg
Phosphorus	47 mg
Protein	3 g
Sodium	57 mg

Lemon Blueberry Corn muffins

Prep time – 10 min

Cook time – 25 min

Total time – 35 min

Ingredients:

(12 servings)

- Yellow cornmeal (¾ cup)
- Whole wheat flour (¾ cup)
- Baking powder (1 ½ teaspoons)
- Granulated sugar (¼ cup)
- Rice milk (¾ cup)
- Melted unsalted butter (2 tablespoons)
- Egg (1)
- Lemon juice (2 tablespoons)
- Lemon zest (1 teaspoon)
- Fresh blueberries (a cup)

Instruction:

- Preheat your oven to 400 degrees.
- Spray your muffin pan with non-stick cooking spray. You can also use an 8 by 8 baking pan.
- Put the cornmeal, baking powder, flour, and sugar in a large mixing bowl.
- Mix the oil or butter, milk, egg, lemon zest, and lemon juice in a smaller bowl.
- Add the wet mixture to the dry mixture and stir until just barely mixed. It is alright to have some lumps.

- Gently stir in the blueberries to the mixture. If using frozen berries, ensure to rinse them with cold water and pat try before you add to the mixture.
- Pour the batter into the muffin pan.
- Bake for approximately 15 minutes if using muffins, or for 25 minutes if baking with the 8 by 8 pan.
- Once ready, drizzle with honey if you want.

Nutrition Facts:

For 12 servings per recipe.

Calories 117

Carbohydrates 19 g

Dietary Fiber 3 g

Potassium 92 mg

Phosphorus 71 mg

Protein 3 g

Fat 2 g

Sodium 76 mg

Strawberry Sorbet - Beverages

Prep time – 5 min

Total time – 5 min

Ingredients:

(3 servings)

- Sugar (¼ cup)
- Fresh or frozen strawberries (1 cup)
- Lemon juice (1 tablespoon)
- Water (¼ cup)
- Cubed or Crushed ice (1 ¼ cups)

Instructions:

- Put the ice in a blender and blend on high speed to crush the ice
- Add all the other ingredients into the blender and blend on high speed
- Serve!

Nutritional facts:

Calories.   67

Carbohydrate. 21 g

Fiber 1 g

Sodium.   1 mg

Potassium.   79 mg

Phosphorus.   12 mg

Cranberry Punch (Beverages)

Prep time – 5 min

Total time – 5 min

Ingredients:

(46 servings)

- Cranberry juice - 3 quarts

- Pineapple juice - 3 quarts

- Undiluted Lemonade - 3 quarts (frozen)

- Water - 1 quart

- A 28-ounce bottle of Ginger ale – 3

Instructions:

- Mix all ingredients in a large jar.

- Refrigerate to cool before serving.

Nutritional facts:

Calories   130

Protein   1 g

Carbohydrate 34 g

Sodium   8 mg

Potassium   153 mg

Phosphorus   16 mg

Russian Tea - Beverages

Yield: 88 serving

Ingredients

- Tang (2 cups)
- Sugar (½ cup)
- One dry lemonade mix
- Instant tea (1 cup)
- Cinnamon (1 teaspoon)
- Cloves (1 teaspoon)

Instructions

- Mix all the ingredients.
- Store the mixture in a covered container.
- To drink, add a tablespoon of the mixture to 8 ounces of hot water.
- Drink hot.

Nutritional facts:

Calories 54

Carbohydrates   13 g

Phosphorus   17 mg

Potassium   25 mg

CHAPTER 3: LUNCH RECIPES

Chicken Tacos

Prep time – 10 min

Cook time – 30 min

Total time – 40 min

Ingredients:

(4 servings)

- Boneless, skinless chicken breast (1 pound)
- Salt-free taco seasoning (1 ½ teaspoon)
- Lime – 1 (juiced)
- Corn tortillas (8)
- Sour cream (¼ cup)
- Iceberg lettuce – 1 (Chopped or shredded)
- green onions – 2 (Sliced)
- cilantro – ½ cup (chopped)

Instruction:

- Boil the chicken for approximately 20 minutes.
- Chop the chicken finely or shred into biteable sizes.
- Toss the chicken along with the lime juice and Mexican seasoning.

- Fill the corn tortillas with lettuce and chicken.

- Topping is optional. You can use the sour cream, cilantro, green onions, or other garnishes for topping.

Nutritional facts:

For four servings per recipe.

Calories   141

Carbohydrates   9 g

Protein   14 g

Sodium   50 mg

Potassium   220 mg

Phosphorus   155 mg

Cucumber & Cream Cheese

Ingredients:

(2 servings)

- cucumber – 1 (remove the seeds and grate)

- 3-ounces Packaged cream cheese – 1 (softened)

- Grated onion (2 tablespoons)

- Tabasco sauce (a dash)

- Mayonnaise (1 tablespoon)

Instructions:

- Mix the ingredients using a blender.

- Spread the mixture on unsalted crackers or bread.

- Garnish with slices of green pepper or paprika.

Nutritional facts:

For two servings per recipe

Calories.   219

Carbohydrates.   48 mg

Dietary fibers.   1 g

Phosphorus.   80 mg

Potassium.   264 mg

Protein.   4 g

Sodium.   185 mg

Party Mix

Ingredients:

(12 servings)

- Corn Chex cereal (2 cups)

- Wheat Chex cereal (2 cups)

- Rice Chex cereal (2 cups)

- Margarine (½ cup)

- Garlic powder (¼ teaspoon)

- Onion powder (¼ teaspoon)

Instructions:

- Preheat your oven to 325 degrees.

- Melt the butter, then add in the cereals and spices. Mix until properly coated.

- Spread mixture on a large baking sheet.

- Bake for approximately 30 minutes or until crunchy, stirring occasionally.

Nutritional facts:

For 12 servings per recipe

Calories. 92

Carbohydrates.   17 g

Dietary fibers. 1 g

Phosphorus.   42 mg

Potassium.   58 mg

Protein. 2 g

Sodium.   349 mg

Deviled Eggs

Prep time – 20 min

Cook time: 15 min

Total time – 35 min

Ingredients:

(1 serving)

- Hard-boiled egg (1)
- Pimentos (1 teaspoon)
- Mayonnaise (1 tablespoon)
- Dry mustard (¼ teaspoon)
- Black pepper (¼ teaspoon)
- paprika (for garnishing)

Instructions:

- Cut the egg into two halves and remove the yolk.
- Mix the pimentos, egg yolk, mayonnaise, dry mustard, and black pepper in a bowl.
- Spoon the mixture into the halved egg whites in equal parts.
- Sprinkle eggs with paprika, if you like.

Nutritional facts:

For one serving per recipe

Calories   116

Carbohydrates.   4 g

Phosphorus.   95 mg

Potassium.   83 mg

Protein.   7 g

Sodium.   78 mg

CHAPTER 4: MAIN DISH RECIPES

Turkey and Noodles

Prep time – 10 min

Cook time – 10 min

Total time – 20 min

Yield – 8 Servings

Ingredients:

- Dry elbow macaroni (2 cups)
- fresh lean ground turkey (2 pounds)
- Olive or vegetable oil (1 tablespoon)
- chopped green onions, (½ cup)
- chopped green pepper (½ cup)
- 14-ounce canned, regular diced tomatoes(1)
- black pepper (1 teaspoon)
- Italian seasoning (1 tablespoon)

Instructions:

- Pour 4 cups of boiling water in a medium boiler and cook the macaroni for about 5 minutes or until tender.
- Then drain the water and keep aside.

- Heat up the vegetable oil in a big frypan over medium heat. Add the ground turkey to the oil and cook until its properly done while you stir occasionally.
- Throw in the cooked macaroni, green peppers, onions, diced tomatoes, black pepper, and Italian seasoning. Mix well.
- Cover the pan and allow to simmer for about 5 minutes.
- Serve warm.

Nutritional facts:

Calories. 273

Protein. 33 g

Carbohydrates. 22 g

Dietary fiber. 2 g

Sodium. 188 mg

Potassium.   533 mg

Phosphorus. 296 mg

Eggplant Casserole

Prep time – 10 min

Cook time – 45 min

Total time – 55 min

Ingredients

(8 servings)

- Large eggplant (1)
- Lean ground turkey or beef (1 pound)
- Vegetable oil - 2 tablespoons (chopped)
- Plain bread crumbs (2 cups)
- green pepper - ½ cup (Chopped)
- onion - ½ cup (Chopped)
- large egg – 1 (slightly beaten)
- Red pepper - ½ teaspoon (optional)

Instructions

- Preheat your oven to 350 degrees.
- Boil the eggplant until it is tender, then drain and mash it
- Heat up the oil, then add the ground meat, onion, and green pepper. Sauté until cooked.
- Add the bread crumbs, eggplant, and egg. Mix well.

- Add red pepper to taste, if you want.

- Place in a casserole dish and bake for approximately 45 minutes.

- Serve warm

Nutritional facts

Calories.   240

Carbohydrates. 5 g

Dietary fibers.   4 g

Protein.   15 g

Sodium.   263 mg

Basic Meat Loaf

Prep time – 15 min

Cook time – 45 min

Total time – 1 hour

Yield – 8 servings

Ingredients:

- Lean ground turkey (1 pound)

- Egg white (1)

- Lemon juice (1 tablespoon)

- Plain bread crumbs (½ cup)

- Onion powder (½ teaspoon)

- Italian seasoning (½ teaspoon)

- Black pepper (¼ teaspoon)

- onions – ½ cup (chopped)

- green bell pepper - ½ cup (diced)

- Water (¼ cup)

Instructions:

- Preheat your oven to 400 degrees.

- Pour the lemon juice over the ground turkey

- Mix the remaining ingredients in a different bowl.

- Add the mixture to the turkey and mix thoroughly.

- Pour the mixture in a loaf pan and bake for approximately 45 minutes.

Nutritional facts:

Calories.   110

Carbohydrates. 2 g

Phosphorus.   87 mg

Potassium.   138 mg

Protein.   12 g

Sodium.   71 mg

Seafood Supreme

Prep time – 10 min

Cook time – 30 min

Total time – 40 min

Yield – 6 Servings

Ingredients

- Bread crumbs - 1 cup
- Crabmeat - 1 cup (cooked/ boiled)
- Shrimp - 1 cup (cooked/ boiled)
- Celery – 1 cup (chopped)
- Green pepper – 4 tablespoons (chopped)
- Green onions – 2 tablespoons (chopped)
- Frozen green peas - ½ cup
- Black pepper - ½ teaspoon
- Mayonnaise - ½ cup

Instructions:

- Preheat your oven to 375 degrees
- Mix all the ingredients, except the bread crumbs, in a medium-sized bowl.
- Put the mixture in an already greased casserole dish.

- Sprinkle with bread crumbs.

- Bake for 30 minutes in the preheated oven

Nutritional facts:

Calories.   222

Carbohydrates. 20 g

Dietary fibers.   2 g

Phosphorus.   148 mg

Potassium.   255 mg

Protein.   16 g

Sodium   445 mg

Crab Cakes

Prep time – 5 min

Cook time – 10 min

Total time – 15 min

Yield – 6 servings

Ingredients:

- One egg

- Finely chopped red or green pepper (1/3 cup)

- Low sodium crackers (1/3 cup)

- Low fat mayonnaise (¼ cup)

- Dry mustard (1 tablespoon)
- Crushed red or black pepper (1 teaspoon)
- Lemon juice (2 tablespoons)
- Garlic powder (1 teaspoon)
- Vegetable oil (2 tablespoons)

Instructions:

- Mix all the ingredients in a bowl
- Divide the mixture into six balls and shape into patties
- Heat the vegetable oil in the oven at 350 degrees, or in a frypan at medium heat.
- Fry or bake the patties; 5 minutes for frying or 15 minutes in the oven

Nutritional facts:

Calories.   101

Carbohydrates.   5 g

Phosphorus.   43 mg

Potassium. 72 mg

Protein. 2 g

Sodium.   67 mg

Chicken'N Rice

Prep time – 20 min

Cook time – 25 min

Total time – 45 min

Yield – 6 servings

Ingredients:

- Chicken parts - 1 pound
- Uncooked rice (1 cup)
- Chopped onion (½ cup)
- Black pepper (1 teaspoon)
- Poultry seasoning (1 tablespoon)
- onion powder - 1 teaspoon
- Garlic powder (½ teaspoon)
- crushed bay leaves - 1 teaspoon (optional)
- water – 4 cups
- Vegetable oil (1 tablespoon)

Instructions:

- Put the bay leaves, chicken part, poultry seasoning, black pepper, onion powder, onions, and garlic powder into a dutch oven; cover with water.

- Cook until the chicken is tender.
- Debone the chicken and discard the skin. Reserve 2 cups of the chicken broth as well as the chicken meat.
- Put the 2 cups of broth, vegetable oil, rice, and chicken in a large pot and allow to boil over medium-high heat.
- Reduce the heat and allow it to cook for approximately 25 minutes.
- Serve hot.

Nutritional facts:

Calories.   212

Carbohydrates.   11 g

Dietary fibers. 1 g

Phosphorus.   218 mg

Potassium.   283 mg

Protein. 21 g

Sodium.   76 mg

Beef & Vegetable Soup

Prep time – 10 min

Cook time – 50 min

Total time – 1 hour

Yield – 8 Servings

Ingredients:

- Beef stew (1 pound)
- Raw sliced onions (1 cup)
- Black pepper (1 teaspoon)
- Thyme (½ teaspoons)
- Basil (½ teaspoon)
- Frozen green peas (½ cup)
- Frozen okra (½ cup)
- Water – 3 ½ cups
- Diced frozen carrots (½ cup)
- Frozen corn (½ cup)

Instructions:

- Place the beef stew, black pepper, water, thyme, basil, and onions in a large pot and cook for approximately 45 minutes.
- Then add all the frozen vegetables; simmer on low heat until the meat is tender. Serve hot.

Note: if the soup requires additional water, add ½ cup per time until you get the desired consistency.

Nutritional facts:

Calories.   190

Carbohydrates.   7 g

Dietary fibers.   2 g

Phosphorus.   121 mg

Potassium.   291 mg

Protein.   11 g

Sodium.   56 mg

Herbed Omelet

Prep time – 10 min

Cook time – 5 min

Total time – 15 min

Ingredients:

(2 servings)

- Vegetable oil (1 ½ teaspoons)
- Eggs - 4
- Chopped onion (1 tablespoon)
- Water – 2 tablespoons
- Tarragon – 1/8 teaspoon
- Basil – ¼ teaspoon
- Parsley – ¼ teaspoon (optional)

Instructions:

- Beat eggs in a bowl, add the spices and water.

- Heat oil in a frypan over medium heat, then add the onions and sauté. Remove the onions from the pan once sautéed.

- Pour the egg mixture into the heated frypan over medium heat.

- While the omelet is cooking, use a spatula to push the cooked part to the middle to let the uncooked portion of the egg flow to the edges.

- Once the omelet is set, spread the sautéed onion on top of the omelet and remove from heat.

- Serve warm.

Nutritional facts:

Calories.   195

Phosphorus.   224 mg

Potassium.   157 mg

Protein.   14 g

Sodium   157 mg

Steak and Onion Sandwich

Prep time – 5 min

Cook time – 10 min

Total time – 15 min

Ingredients:

(4 servings)

- chopped steaks (4 pieces of 4-ounces each)
- Hoagie rolls – 4 (sliced)
- Lemon juice (1 tablespoon)
- Sliced onion (1 medium bulb)
- Italian seasoning (1 tablespoon)
- Black pepper (1 tablespoon)
- Vegetable oil (1 tablespoon)

Instructions:

- Put the meat in a bowl, add the lemon juice, black pepper, and Italian seasoning, then mix properly.
- Heat the vegetable oil in a frypan over medium heat.
- Cook the steaks for about 3 minutes, until they are brown on both sides and tender.
- Place the steaks on paper towels to drain.
- Put the onion in the frypan and sauté under low heat until the onions get tender
- Serve the steak on the hoagie rolls and top with the onion rings

Nutritional facts:

For four servings per recipe

Calories   345

Carbohydrates.   26 g

Dietary fibers   2 g

Phosphorus.   115 mg

Potassium   200 mg

Protein   14 g

Sodium   247 mg

Taco Stuffing

Prep time – 5 min

Cook time – 5 min

Total time – 10 min

Ingredients:

(8 servings)

- Lean ground turkey or beef (1 ¼ pounds)
- Shredded lettuce (½ head)
- Vegetable oil (2 tablespoons)
- Ground black pepper (½ teaspoon)
- Ground red pepper (½ teaspoon)

- Italian seasoning (1 teaspoon)

- Onion powder (1 teaspoon)

- Garlic powder (1 teaspoon)

- Tabasco sauce (½ teaspoon)

- Nutmeg (½ teaspoon)

- medium-sized Taco shells – 1

Instructions:

- Heat the oil over medium heat.

- Place all the ingredients, minus the lettuce and taco shells, in a skillet.

- Cook the beef till its done, and all the ingredients are properly blended.

- Stuff the taco shells with approximately two ounces of meat or turkey.

- Add the shredded lettuce as a topping.

Nutritional facts:

For eight servings per recipe

Calories.   176

Carbohydrates. 9 g

Phosphorus.   33 mg

Potassium.   258 mg

Protein.   14 g

Sodium.   124 mg

Barbecue cups

Prep time – 3 min

Cook time – 12 min

Total time – 15 min

Ingredients:

(10 servings)

- Lean ground turkey (¾ pounds)
- Low-fat refrigerator biscuits - 1 10-ounces package
- Spicy barbecue sauce (½ cup)
- Garlic powder (a dash)
- Onion flakes (2 teaspoons)
- Olive oil (2 tablespoons)

Instructions:

- Grease a pan with olive oil and heat over medium heat.
- Place the ground turkey in the greased pan and cook until it's brown on both sides (flip to the other side to get it browned).
- Add the onion flakes, barbecue sauce, and garlic powder and mix properly.
- Press the biscuit into the muffin tins.

- Scoop the beef mixture into the middle of the individual biscuit cups.
- Bake at 400 degrees F for approximately 12 minutes.

Nutritional facts:

calories. 134

Carbohydrates.   13 g

Phosphorus.   152 mg

Potassium.   151 mg

Protein. 7 g

Sodium.   342 mg

Seafood Croquettes

Prep time – 5 min

Cook time – 5 min

Total time – 10 min

Ingredients:

(8 servings)

- Fresh or frozen crab meat (1 pound) or water-packed tuna or salmon – 1 can
- Unsalted cracker crumbs (½ cup)

- Egg whites (2)

- Chopped onion (¼ cup)

- Regular mayonnaise – ¼ cup (crab and tuna only)

- Black pepper (½ teaspoon)

- Cooking spray or Vegetable oil (1 tablespoon)

- Ground mustard – ½ teaspoon (crab only)

- Lemon juice (2 tablespoons)

Instructions:

- Remove the water from the canned meat.

- Add all the ingredients in a medium-sized bowl, minus the oil. Mix them well.

- Make eight separate balls from the mixture and shape to form patties.

- Put the vegetable oil in a pan and heat it.

- Once the oil gets hot, place the patties in the pan.

- Allow the patties to get brown on each side.

- Place the patties on a paper towel to drain if soaked in oil.

Nutritional facts:

For eight servings per recipe

Calories. 189

Carbohydrates. 11 g

Dietary fibers. 1 g

Phosphorus.   191 mg

 Protein.   14 g

Sodium   337 mg

Shrimp Salad

Ingredients:

(4 servings)

- Shrimp (1 pound)
- Hard-boiled egg – 1 (chopped)
- Green pepper - 2 tablespoons (chopped)
- Celery - 1 teaspoon (chopped)
- Onion - 1 tablespoon (chopped)
- Mayonnaise - 2 tablespoons
- Chili powder (½ teaspoon)
- Lemon juice (1 teaspoon)
- Dry mustard (½ teaspoon)
- Hot sauce or Tabasco (1/8 teaspoon)
- Shredded or chopped lettuce - a handful (optional)

Instructions:

- Boil, chop and devein the shrimps.
- Mix all ingredients in a bowl (excluding the lettuce).
- Keep in the refrigerator to cool for 30 minutes.
- Serve on a sandwich or a salad. Add the chopped lettuce, if desired.

Nutritional Facts:

Calories.   157

Carbohydrates.   1 g

Phosphorus   263 mg

Potassium.   233 m

Protein.   26 g

Sodium   232 mg

Fish Tacos

Prep time – 5 min

Cook time – 10 min

Total time – 15 min

Ingredients:

(4 servings)

- 1 pound of your preferred fish fillets – 12 to 16

- Unsalted crackers or tops – 20 (crush finely)
- Unsalted margarine or butter (¼ cup)
- Dill weed (2 teaspoons)
- Garlic powder (1 teaspoon)
- Lemon juice (¼ cup)

Instructions:

- Preheat your oven to 400 degrees.
- Mix the crackers, dill, and garlic.
- Melt the margarine or butter.
- Roll fish in melted margarine or butter, then roll in the crumbs mix before rolling again in the butter mix.
- Place the fish in a baking pan and bake for approximately 10 minutes or until the fish is flakey.

Nutritional facts:

For four servings per recipe

Calories.   164

Carbohydrates. 7 g

Phosphorus.   181 mg

Potassium.   335 mg

Protein. 21 g

Sodium.   138 mg

Special Pizza

Prep time – 25 min

Cook time – 35 min

Total time – 1 hour

Ingredients:

For crust

(10 slices)

- All-purpose flour (2 cups)

- Granulated sugar (1 tablespoon)

- Active dry yeast (1 teaspoon)

- Water (1 cup)

- Vegetable shortening (2 tablespoons)

Instructions:

For crust

- Mix the yeast, flour, and sugar in a large bowl

- Add the vegetable shortening to the dry ingredients and use a fork to mix all the ingredients.

- Add water little by little as you mix with the fork until the mixture moves freely with the fork around the bowl.

- Cover the dough and allow it to rest for approximately 15 minutes.

Ingredients for pizza topping:

- low-fat sharp cheddar cheese - 4 ounces (Grated)
- Ground lean chicken, turkey or beef (½ pound)
- Italian seasoning (1 ½ teaspoons)
- Onion powder (½ teaspoon)
- Garlic powder (½ teaspoon)
- Chilli powder (1 teaspoon)
- Tomato paste (¼ cup)
- Vegetable oil (½ cup)
- Diced onions (½ cup)
- Diced green peppers (½ cup)

Instructions:

- Preheat your oven to 425 degrees
- Sauté the ground chicken or meat in a frypan.
- Add the onion powder, half teaspoon of Italian seasoning, and garlic powder to the chicken. Continue stirring until the chicken is well cooked.
- Place the beef on a paper towel to drain.

- Get the sauce ready by mixing the chilli powder, tomato paste, remaining Italian seasoning, and water in a bowl. Keep aside.
- After the dough has rested, oil your fingers and the pizza pan.
- Evenly spread the dough on the pan.
- Then spread the sauce evenly over the pizza dough. Sprinkle a half cup of cheese on the pizza.
- Place in the oven to cook for approximately 20 minutes.
- Take out from the oven and add the remaining cheese, ground beef, onions, and green pepper.
- Return the pan to the oven for another 10 minutes.
- Serve hot!

Nutritional facts:

For ten slices per recipe

Calories.   196

Carbohydrates.   24 g

Dietary fibers.   2 g

Phosphorus.   31 mg

Potassium.   188 mg

Protein.   11 g

Sodium.   144 mg

Stuffed Green Peppers

Prep time – 10 min

Cook time – 30 min

Total time – 40 min

Ingredients:

(6 servings)

- Ground lean beef, chicken or turkey (½ pound)
- Cooked rice (1 ½ cups)
- Vegetable oil (2 tablespoons)
- Celery seed (1 tablespoon)
- Chopped onions (¼ cup)
- Chopped celery (¼ cup)
- Italian seasoning (2 tablespoons)
- Lemon juice (2 tablespoons)
- Black pepper (1 tablespoon)
- Sugar (½ teaspoon)
- small green peppers – 6 (deseed and remove the tops)

- Paprika

Instructions:

- Preheat your oven to 325 degrees.
- Heat oil in a saucepan.
- Add onions, ground beef, and celery to the saucepan and cook until the meat turns brown.
- Add the remaining ingredients (except paprika and green peppers) to the saucepan.
- Stir them together, then remove from heat.
- Stuff the mixture into the peppers. Wrap with foil or put them into a dish and cover.
- Place in the oven to bake for approximately 30 minutes.
- Take out of the oven and sprinkle with paprika

Nutritional facts:

For six servings per recipe

Calories. 131

Carbohydrates. 15 g

Dietary fibers. 1 g

Phosphorus. 83 mg

Potassium. 160 mg

Protein. 9 g

Sodium.   36 mg

Fajitas

Prep time – 5 min

Cook time – 22min

Total time – 27 min

Ingredients:

(4 servings)

- Raw chicken or beef strips or shrimps - 1 ½ pound (peeled and deveined)
- Vegetable oil (2 tablespoons)
- Chilli powder (2 teaspoons)
- Lime or lemon juice (2 tablespoons)
- Cumin (½ teaspoon)
- Red and/ or green pepper - ¼ pepper (Sliced lengthwise)
- Dry cilantro - ½ teaspoon
- white onions - ½ bulb (Sliced lengthwise)
- Flour tortillas – 4
- Vegetable spray

Instructions

- Preheat your oven to 300 degrees F.
- Pour the vegetable oil into a non-stick frypan and place over medium heat.
- Add the chicken strips, seasonings, and lime/lemon juice, cook for about 10 minutes or until the meat is tender.
- Add the onion and green pepper to the pan and cook for an additional two minutes.
- Remove the pan from heat and add the cilantro.
- Place tortillas on foil and put in the oven — Cook for approximately 10 minutes.
- Share the mixtures between the tortillas.
- Wrap and serve.

Nutritional facts:

For four servings per recipe

Calories 184

Carbohydrates. 5 g

Dietary fibers. 1 g

Phosphorus.   207 mg

Potassium.   494 mg

Protein. 19 g

Sodium.   121 mg

CHAPTER 5: SIDE DISH RECIPES

Pineapple Coleslaw

Prep time – 5 min

Total time – 5 min

Ingredients:

(4 servings)

- Shredded cabbage (2 cups)
- Crushed unsweetened pineapple (1 - 8-ounce can)
- Red apple (1) - cubed
- Onion (¼ of a cup) - chopped
- Carrot (1) - Grated
- Mayonnaise or miracle whip (¼ cup)

Instruction:

- Put all the ingredients in a bowl and mix until everything is coated.
- Keep in the refrigerator for at least 1 hour before serving.

Nutritional facts:

For four servings per recipe

Calories   128

Carbohydrates   8 g

Phosphorus.   14 mg

Potassium.   143 mg

Protein   1 g

Sodium   81 mg

Old Fashioned Pancakes

Prep time- 5 min

Cook time- 5 min

Total time- 10 min

Yield: 4 small pancakes

Ingredients:

- All-purpose flour (½ cup)
- Baking powder (¼ teaspoon)
- Egg – 1 (beaten)
- Granulated sugar (¼ cup)
- Water (¼ cup)
- 2% milk (¼ cup)
- Vegetable oil (1 tablespoon)

Instructions:

- Mix the flour, egg, sugar, and baking powder in a bowl then add water and milk. Add less water if you want thick pancakes or more water if you want slimmer pancakes.

- Heat oil on a griddle or in a pan and scoop ¼ cup of batter into the pan. Cook until the pancake turns brown on each side.

Nutritional facts:

Calories. 165

Carbohydrates.   26 g

Phosphorus.   64 mg

Potassium. 57 mg

Sodium.   58 mg

Macaroni Salad

Prep time – 10 min

Total time – 10 min

Ingredients:

(8 servings)

- hard-boiled eggs - 3 (shelled and Chopped)
- Cooked Macaroni (3 cups)
- Pimentos (¼ cup)
- green pepper - ½ cup (Chopped)
- Onion – ½ cup (Chopped)

- Mayonnaise (½ cup)

- Celery – ½ cup (Chopped)

- Black pepper

- Dry mustard (1 teaspoon)

- Paprika

Instructions:

- Rinse the cooked macaroni under cold running water and drain well.

- Add the remaining ingredients (except the black pepper and paprika) to the macaroni and mix well.

- Sprinkle the black pepper and paprika.

- Serve chilled

Nutritional facts:

For eight servings per recipe

Calories   223

Carbohydrates. 18 g

Phosphorus. 74 mg

Potassium   106 mg

Protein. 6 g

Sodium.   103 mg

Marinated Vegetables

Prep time – 10 min

Total time- 10 min

Yield: 15 serving

Ingredients for marinade

- Vinegar - ¾ cup
- Sugar - ¾ cup
- Water - 1 tablespoon
- Black pepper (to taste)

Ingredient for salad

- 12-ounce can of shoe peg corn – 1 (drained)
- 12-ounce can of English peas – 1 (drained)
- A 12-ounce jar of Pimento - 1 (drained)
- celery – 1 cup (finely chopped)
- onion – ¾ cup (finely chopped)

Instructions:

- Mix all the marinade ingredients in a small cooking pot and bring to a boil. Allow to cool completely.
- Toss the salad ingredients together.
- Pour the marinade over the salad and stir.
- Refrigerate overnight before serving.

Note: If you are not able to find shoe peg corn, you can use yellow or white corn.

Nutritional facts:

Calories. 85

Carbohydrates. 20 g

Dietary fibers. 2 g

Phosphorus. 39 mg

Potassium. 154 mg

Protein. 1 g

Sodium. 13 mg

Vegetables & Rice

Prep time – 5 min

Cook time – 10 min

Total time – 15 min

Ingredients:

(6 servings)

- Cooked salt-free rice (2 ½ cups)
- 10-ounce frozen green peas – 1 (cook and drain the water)

- Medium-sized onion – 1 (chopped)

- Unsalted Margarine – ¼ cup

- Lemon juice – 1 tablespoon

- Thyme – ½ teaspoon

- Liquid smoke, optional – 2 tablespoons

Instructions

- Sauté the chopped onion in margarine until it's tender.

- Add the rice, lemon juice, thyme, green peas, and liquid smoke.

- Cook for approximately 5 minutes.

Nutritional facts:

Calories. 194

Carbohydrates. 26

Dietary fibers. 3 g

Phosphorus. 67 mg

Potassium. 99 mg

Protein. 4 g

Sodium. 32 mg

Healthy Chips

Ingredients

(4 servings)

- Potatoes (908 g)
- A small amount of olive oil, spray oil or vegetable oil

Instruction:

- Preheat your oven to 240 degrees
- Peel and slice the potatoes lengthwise to about half-inch thick rectangular chips.
- Add water to a large pot, add salt, bring to a boil.
- Then add the chips and cook for approximately 4 minutes.
- Drain the water and keep aside for 10 minutes to dry.
- Place the chips in a dry pot, cover with a lid, then shake the pot to roughen the edges of the chips.
- Lightly grease a metal baking tray with spray or olive oil.
- Move the chips to the tray, spray lightly with oil spray or apply olive oil lightly on the chips.

- Place pan in the oven and bake for about 20 to 25 minutes, occasionally turning until the chips turn golden brown on all sides.
- Place them on a kitchen paper to drain before you serve.

CHAPTER 6: DINNER RECIPES

Egg Salad

Total time – 5 min

Yield – 8 servings

Ingredients:

- Mayonnaise (2 tablespoons)
- Dry mustard (1 teaspoon)
- Black pepper (½ teaspoon)
- boiled eggs – 3 (Chopped)
- Pickle relish (1 tablespoon)
- Paprika

Instructions:

- Mix all the ingredients (minus the paprika) in a bowl
- Sprinkle the paprika over the mixture

Nutritional facts:

Calories   58

Carbohydrates. 1 g

Phosphorus.   36 mg

Potassium. 28 mg

Protein. 3 g

Sodium   58 mg

Baked Potato Soup

Prep time- 10 min

Cook time – 10 min

Total time – 20 min

Ingredients:

(6 servings)

- Potatoes (2)
- Flour - 1/3 cup
- Skimmed milk - 4 cups
- Pepper (½ teaspoon)
- Low-fat Monterey jack cheese - 4 ounces (shredded)
- Fat-free sour cream (½ cup)

Instruction:

- Bake the potatoes in the oven until they are tender at 400 degrees F.
- Allow the potatoes to cool, then cut in half and take out the pulp.
- Spread flour in a large pot and slowly add milk, stir until blended.
- Add pepper and the potato pulp to the large pot.

- Cook the mixture over medium heat until it becomes thick and bubbly. Remember to stir frequently.
- Add cheese to the pot and stir until melted.
- Remove the mixture from heat and stir in your sour cream.

Nutritional facts:

Calories   216

Carbohydrates   29 g

Dietary Fiber 4 g

Potassium   594 mg

Phosphorus   326 mg

Protein   15 g

Sodium   272 mg

Stir fry Meal

Prep time – 10 min

Cook time – 10 min

Total time – 20 min

Ingredients:

(2 servings)

- Mixed greens of your choice – 4 cups (beet, collard, lettuce, etc.)
- Olive oil - 1 tablespoon
- Sliced onions (1 cup)
- Curry powder - ¼ teaspoon
- Low sodium soy sauce - 1 tablespoon
- Rice vinegar or white wine vinegar (½ cup)
- Cubed tofu (8 ounces)
- Sesame oil (½ teaspoon)
- Sesame seeds (½ teaspoon)

Instruction:

- Cut the greens into long shreds or as desired
- Heat oil in a sauté pan or a wok.
- Sauté the onions for about 2 minutes, until translucent.
- Sprinkle curry on the onions then add the greens and sugar.
- Cover the pan.
- Reduce to low heat and steam the greens in its juice until tender. This should take about 6 to 8 minutes. While cooking, turn occasionally. Add a little water if needed.

- Use a slotted spoon to remove the greens and leave the juice in the pan.
- Add vinegar and soy sauce to the juice and allow it to boil.
- When the juice becomes slightly thick, take the pan off the heat and pour over the greens.
- Garnish with sesame seeds and oil.

Nutrition Facts Based on two servings per recipe.

Calories   231

Carbohydrates   13 g

Protein   14 g

Sodium   355 mg

Potassium   442 mg

Phosphorus   54 mg

Paella

Prep time – 10 min

Cook time – 20 min

Total time – 30 min

Ingredients:

(8 servings)

- Olive oil (1 tablespoon)

- Italian sausage (½ pound)
- Diced chicken breast (½ pound)
- Pressed garlic (2 cloves)
- Uncooked short-grain rice (2 cups)
- Chopped yellow onion (1 cup)
- Low sodium chicken broth (1 ½ cup)
- Roasted red peppers - 2 jars (pureed)
- Paprika (½ teaspoon)
- Tabasco sauce (½ teaspoon)
- Saffron - 1/8 teaspoon or ten strands
- Shrimp - ½ pound (shelled, deveined, uncooked)
- red pepper – ½ cup (sliced)
- Green peppers – ½ cup (sliced)
- Frozen green pea – ½ cup (sliced)

Instruction:

- Heat olive oil in large sauté pan and sauté the chicken, sausage, and garlic until the chicken turns brown.
- Remove the meats and keep aside.
- Add onion and rice to the sauté pan and sauté until the rice is golden brown and the onion is translucent.

- Add the meats to the frypan along with the pureed red bell peppers and the meat broth.
- Add the Tabasco, paprika, and saffron.
- Allow to boil, then reduce the heat and leave to simmer for approximately 10 minutes.
- Add the bell peppers, shrimp, and peas and stir.
- Cook for another 10 minutes

Nutritional Facts:

Calories   233

Carbohydrates   25 g

Protein   20 g

Dietary Fiber 6 g

Sodium   257 mg

Potassium   330 mg

Phosphorus   201 mg

Chicken nuggets

Prep time – 5 min

Cook time – 15 min

Total time – 20 min

Ingredients:

(4 servings)

- Skinless, boneless chicken breasts - 2
- Dijon mustard (¼ cup)
- Panko bread crumbs (1 cup)

Instruction:

- Preheat your oven to 500 degrees.
- Dry the chicken with a towel, then cut into biteable nugget sizes.
- Dredge the chicken in Dijon mustard and roll in the bread crumbs.
- Place the chicken on a baking sheet and bake for approximately 15 minutes

Nutritional facts:

Calories   247

Carbohydrates   20 g

Protein   31 g

Dietary Fiber 3 g

Sodium   484 mg

Potassium   384 mg

Phosphorus   284 mg

Fiesta Lime Tacos

Prep time – 5 min

Cook time – 15 min

Total time – 20 min

Ingredients

(12 servings)

- Mrs. Dash Fiesta Lime Seasoning blend (4 tablespoons)
- Lean ground turkey or beef (1 pound)
- Water (¾ cup)
- Taco shells (12)

Instructions

- Cook the ground beef over medium-high heat until browned.
- Drain excess fat.
- Add in lime seasoning blend and water. Stir.
- Allow to boil, then reduce the heat and allow to simmer for 5 minutes while stirring occasionally.
- Scoop the mixture into warm taco shells.
- Serve with any toppings of your choice.

Nutritional facts:

Calories 140

Carbohydrates. 9 g

Dietary fibers.   1 g

Phosphorus.   111 mg

Potassium.   140 mg

Protein.   7 g

Sodium.   70 mg

Fish Pie

Prep Time: 5 mins

Cook Time: 40 mins

Total Time: 45 mins

Ingredients:

(4 servings)

- Swede (300 g)

- Potatoes (300 g)

- Vegetable oil (1 tablespoon)

- Mixed herbs (1 teaspoon)

- Chopped onion (1)

- Fish pie mix (600 g)

- Semi-skimmed milk (75 ml)

- Cream cheese (200 g)

- Grated cheddar cheese (20 g)

Instruction:

- Cook the Swede and potatoes in a pot of boiling water until soft. Drain the water and keep aside.

- Heat up the oil in a non-stick skillet and add the herbs and onion. Cook until the onion is tender.

- Add the fish to the skillet and cook until the fish is well cooked. Add the cream cheese and stir until the cream cheese melts and is bubbly. Add in the milk gradually.

- Add pepper to taste.

- Scoop the fish mixture into an oven-proof dish.

- Add the drained mashed potatoes and swede to the fish mixture. Sprinkle the grated cheese on top and place in the oven for 5 minutes, until the cheese melts.

Turkey and Apple Curry

Ingredients:

- Turkey (500 g)

- Rice milk (1 cup)

- Medium apples (2)

- Black pepper (½ a teaspoon)

- Minced garlic (1 clove)

* Butter (3 tablespoons)

* Dried basil (½ a tablespoon)

* Curry powder (1 tablespoon)

* All-purpose flour (1 tablespoon)

* Low sodium chicken stock (1 cup)

* A handful of fresh coriander

Instruction:

* Heat your oven to 180 degrees.

* Mix the apple, onion, garlic, and butter in a saucepan and cook over medium heat.

* Add the basil and curry powder to the saucepan, mix well and cook for a minute.

* Stir in the flour, continue to cook for another one minute.

* Pour in the rice milk and chicken stock, stir well. Remove the saucepan from heat.

* Add the turkey and coriander and heat again until very hot.

Nutritional facts:

Calories. 380

Sodium.   638 mg

carbohydrate   20 g

protein.   29 g

CHAPTER 7: DESSERT RECIPES

Jewelled Cookies

Prep time – 10 min

Cook time – 20 min (minus chill time)

Total time – 30 min

Ingredients:

(50 cookies)

- Softened unsalted margarine or butter (½ a cup)
- Sifted all-purpose flour (1 ¾ cup)
- Brown sugar - 1 cup (packed)
- Medium egg (1)
- Vanilla (1 teaspoon)
- Milk (¼ cup)
- Baking powder (1 teaspoon)
- Large gumdrops – 15 (chopped)

Instructions:

- Preheat your oven to 400 degrees.
- Mix the egg, butter, and sugar thoroughly in a bowl.
- Add in vanilla and milk, then stir.
- Mix the flour and baking powder together in a different bowl. Add to the previous mixture.

- Now add the gumdrops and stir, then chill for a minimum of one hour.
- Scoop the dough using a tablespoon and place on an oiled cookie sheet.
- Bake for approximately 10 minutes or until it turns golden brown.

Nutritional facts:

calories.   104

protein. 1 g

carbohydrate.   22 g

sodium.   9 mg

potassium.   29 mg

phosphorus.   16 mg

Cream Cheese Cookies

Prep time – 10 min

Cook time – 15 min

Total time – 25 min

Ingredients

(7 dozen cookies)

- 3-ounce package cream cheese – 1 (softened)

- Softened margarine or butter (1 cup)

- Sugar - 1 cup

- Egg yolk – 1

- Vanilla extract (1 teaspoon)

- All-purpose flour (2 ½ cups)

- Candied cherry halves

Instructions:

- Preheat your oven to 325 degrees.

- Mix the cream cheese and butter together, then gradually add sugar, beating as you add until the mixture becomes fluffy.

- Add the egg yolk to the mixture and beat; then add vanilla and flour. Mix well.

- Refrigerate the dough for at least an hour.

- Mold the dough into 1-inch balls and place them on an oiled cookie sheet.

- Gently press a cherry half into each of the cookies.

- Bake for approximately 15 minutes.

Nutritional facts:

Calories. 80

Protein.   0.5 g

Carbohydrates.   11 g

Sodium.   31 mg

Potassium.   15 mg

phosphorus   14 mg

Frozen Lemon Dessert

Prep time – 10 min

Total time – 10 min (minus chill time)

Ingredients:

- Eggs – 4 (Separated)

- Lemon juice (¼ cup)

- Sugar (2/3 cup)

- Lemon peel - 1 tablespoon (Grated)

- Vanilla wafers - 2 cups/ about 40 (Crushed)

- Whipping cream - 1 cup (whipped)

Instructions:

- Beat the egg yolks until it becomes very thick.

- Slowly add sugar and beat each time you add.

- Add the lemon peel and lemon juice, mix well.

- Put the mixture in a double boiler and cook over boiling water, constantly stirring until the mixture gets thick.

- Take off heat and keep aside to cool.

- Beat the egg whites until it forms stiff peaks.

- Fold the egg whites into the thick mixture once cooled.

- Add whipped cream and fold in.

- Spread one and a half crumbs of the vanilla wafer in the bottom of a baking dish or freezer tray.

- Scoop the lemon mixture and spread over the crumbs.

- Sprinkle the remaining vanilla wafer crumbs on the top.

- Freeze for several hours until the mixture is firm.

Nutritional facts:

Calorie. 205

Protein. 3 g

Carbohydrate. 32 g

Sodium.   97 mg

Potassium.   69 mg

Phosphorus.   33 mg

Fruit In The Clouds

Prep time – 10 min

Total time – 10 min

Ingredients:

- Canned fruit cocktail - 1 can (drained)
- Mandarin orange - 1 can (drained)
- Whipped cream - 8 ounces (frozen)

Instructions:

- Put all ingredients in a bowl and mix thoroughly.
- Place mixture into individual moulds or in an 8-inch by 8-inch container. Freeze.
- Serve chilled!

Nutritional facts:

Calories. 113

Protein. 1 g

Carbohydrates. 23 g

Fiber. 2 g

Sodium. 20 mg

Potassium. 152 mg

Phosphorus. 29 mg

Fruit Salad

Prep time – 10 min

Total time – 10 min (Minus chill time)

Ingredients:

(10 servings)

- Canned pineapple chunks – 1 cup (drained)
- Canned fruit cocktail – 2 cups (drained)
- Sliced or whole strawberries – 1 cup (hulled)
- Marshmallows (1 cup)
- Peeled, cored and chopped apple - 1 cup
- Non-diary whipped topping (½ cup)

Instructions:

- Mix all the fruits in a bowl.
- Add the whipped topping and marshmallows. Mix well.
- Refrigerate for at least an hour.
- Serve chilled!

Nutritional facts:

Calories. 57

Protein. 1 g

Carbohydrates.   14 g

 Fiber. 1 g

Sodium. 9 mg

Potassium.   120 mg

 Phosphorus. 15 mg

Blueberry Cobbler

Prep time – 35 min

Cook time – 25 min

Total time – 1 hour

Ingredients for crust:

(10 servings)

- All-purpose flour (1 ½ cups)

- Butter (2 tablespoons)

- Allspice, sugar, and cinnamon (½ a teaspoon)

- Water (¾ cups)

Ingredients for filling:

- 15-ounce Canned blueberries – 1 (packed in light syrup)

- All-purpose flour - 1 cup

- Sugar (½ cup)

- vanilla extract (½ teaspoon)

- A pint of fresh blueberries (rinse and drain)

- A dash of cinnamon

- Margarine or Butter (¼ stick)

Instructions for the crust:

- Mix the butter and the flour together.

- Add water to the mixture, one tablespoon at a time, and mix until the mixture holds together.

- Place the dough on a floured work surface/ top and knead until it is easy to handle (approximately four times).

- Roll out the dough very thinly with a rolling pin or something similar.

- Prepare your filling (refer to the instruction guide).

- Cut the dough into thin strips and place over the filling forming a crisscross pattern

- Sprinkle with sugar, cinnamon and allspice mixture

- Place in the oven to bake for about 20 to 25 minutes or until it turns brown.

Instructions for filing:

- Preheat your oven to 375 degrees.

- Drain the canned berries but reserve ¾ cup of the berry juice.
- Mix the sugar and flour in a pot and add the berry juice you reserved.
- Place the pot over medium heat and stir until the mixture is slightly thick and clear.
- Add the blueberries, vanilla, and cinnamon to the mixture. Mix well.
- Pour the mixture into a deep dish for baking.
- Arrange pieces of butter over the filling.
- Then continue with the steps above.

Nutritional facts:

Calories. 196

Protein.   3 g

Carbohydrate 39 g

Fiber. 3 g

Sodium. 33 mg

Potassium. 76 mg

Phosphorus. 30 mg

Chocolate Pie Shell

Prep time – 40 min

Total time – 40 min

Ingredients:

(6 servings)

- Cocoa Krispies - 3 cups (crushed)
- Butter - 4 tablespoons/ ½ stick
- cooking spray

Instructions:

- Crush the cocoa Krispies, melt the butter and add both to a bowl and stir.
- Spray a 9-inch pie pan with cooking spray, then press the mixture into the pie pan.
- Place in the refrigerator to chill for a minimum of 30 minutes before filling.
- You can add any filling of your choice

Nutritional facts:

Calories. 126

Protein. 2 g

Carbohydrate. 18 g

Sodium. 135 mg

Potassium. 47 mg

Phosphorus. 24 mg

Pumpkin Soufflé

Prep time – 10 min

Cook time – 45 min

Total time – 55 min

Ingredients:

(6 servings)

- Frozen Apple Juice Concentrate - ½ Cup (Do Not Dilute)
- 2 whole eggs/ egg substitute
- 12-ounce canned pumpkin – 1
- Whole milk (1 cup)
- Water (½ cup)
- Ground nutmeg - ½ teaspoon
- Vanilla extract - ½ teaspoon
- Ground allspice - ½ teaspoon
- Grape nuts (½ cup)
- Ground cinnamon (1 teaspoon)
- Pumpkin pie spice - ½ teaspoon (optional)

Instructions:

- Preheat your oven to 400 degrees.

- Put all the ingredients (except grape nuts) into a bowl and mix properly.
- Spray a pie plate with cooking spray and pour the mixture into the plate.
- Spread the grape nuts on top of the mixture.
- Bake for approximately 45 minutes, or until you insert a knife in the center of the pie and it comes out clean.

Nutritional facts:

Calories.   129

Protein. 5 g

Carbohydrate. 26 g

Fiber.   3 g

Sodium.   120 mg

Potassium.   387 mg

Phosphorus.   112 mg

Frozen Fantasy

Prep time – 10 min

Total time – 10 min

Ingredients:

(4 servings)

- Cranberry juice (1 cup)
- Fresh whole strawberries - 1 cup (washed and hulled)
- Fresh lime juice (2 tablespoons)
- sugar (¼ cup)
- ice cubes – 9
- A handful of strawberries for garnish

Instructions:

- Blend the cranberry juice, sugar, lime juice, and strawberries in a blender.
- Blend until the mixture is smooth, then add ice cubes and blend till smooth.
- Pour into a glass and add strawberries to garnish.

Nutritional fact:

For four servings per recipe

Calories. 100

Carbohydrates. 24 g

Dietary fibers. 1 g

Phosphorus. 129 mg

Potassium. 109 mg

Sodium. 3 mg

Ribbon Cakes

Prep time – 10 min

Cook time – 30 min

Total time – 40 min

Serving size: 2 cookies

Ingredients:

- Unsifted all-purpose flour (3 cups)
- Whole eggs (2)
- Sugar (1 cup)
- Baking powder (1 teaspoon)
- Jelly or jam like apricot jam, raspberry jelly, Margarine or butter - 1 cup (Softened)
- Egg white (1)
- Vanilla – ½ teaspoon
- blackberry, or plum - 1 cup
- Sugar – 2 tablespoons

Instructions:

- Heat your oven to 375 degrees.
- Mix the sugar, flour, and baking powder in a bowl.

- Use a pastry blender or your fingertips to blend in the butter until the mixture begins to look like cornmeal.
- Add egg white, eggs, and vanilla into the mixture and work into a stiff dough.
- Divide the dough into two, with one part being twice the size of the other.
- Spread about ¼ to ½ cups of flour on a board and roll out the bigger ball to approximately 1/8 inches thickness.
- Put the rolled dough in a cookie pan and smoothen the edges. Spread the jelly/ jam on the top.
- Roll out the leftover dough to the same thickness and cut into half-inch wide strips.
- Place the strips diagonally across the jam or jelly, half-inch apart.
- Sprinkle sugar over the top of the dough and put it into the oven.
- When the edges begin to brown after about 20 minutes, remove from the oven, and cut off about 3 inches around all the edges.

- Take out the cut-off parts and place the pan back into the oven for approximately 10 minutes.
- Cut into 1-inch by 2-inches rectangles to give you seven dozen cookies.

Nutritional facts:

Calories. 106

Carbohydrates.   15 g

Phosphorus.   27 mg

Potassium.   17 mg

Protein.   1 g

Sodium   65 mg

Baked Egg Custard

Prep time – 10 min

Cook time- 30 min

Total time – 40 min

Ingredients

(4 servings)

- Eggs (2 medium-sized)
- 2% milk (¼ cup)
- Sugar (3 tablespoons)
- Lemon extract or vanilla (1 teaspoon)

- Nutmeg (1 teaspoon)

Instructions

- Preheat your oven to 325 degrees.
- Mix all the ingredients together, use an electric mixer to beat them for one minute until thoroughly mixed.
- Pour the mixture into muffin pans or custard cups.
- Sprinkle a teaspoon of nutmeg on top.
- Bake for approx. 30 minutes. To confirm that the cake is ready, insert a knife in the center of the custard, which should come out clean

Nutritional facts:

Calories. 70

Carbohydrates.   9 g

Phosphorus.   42 mg

Potassium.   30 mg

Protein   3 g

Sodium.   34 mg

Lemon Crispies

Prep time – 10 minutes

Cook time – 10 min

Total time – 10 min

Ingredients

(5 dozen cookies)

- Unsalted margarine or butter (1 cup)
- Egg (1)
- Granulated sugar (1 cup)
- Lemon extract (1 ½ teaspoons)
- All-purpose flour - 1 ½ a cup (sifted)

Instructions

- Preheat your oven to 375 degrees.
- Mix the butter and sugar.
- Add lemon extract and eggs to the mixture and beat until it becomes fluffy and light.
- Add flour to the mixture and beat until smooth.
- Scoop the batter with a tablespoon and place it on an ungreased cookie sheet leaving at least 2-inch space between the cookies.
- Bake for about 10 minutes or until the cookies turn brown around the edges.
- Allow the cookies to cool before you remove them from the cookie sheet

Nutritional facts:

Calories. 115

Carbohydrates. 12 g

Phosphorus. 23 mg

Potassium. 20 mg

Protein. 2 g

Sodium   12 mg

Spritz Cookies

Prep time – 10 min

Cook time – 8 min

Total time – 18 min

Ingredients

(75 cookies)

- All-purpose flour (5 cups)
- Sugar (1 cup + 2 tablespoons)
- Butter (2 cups)
- Eggs (2)
- Almond extract (1 teaspoon)
- Vanilla extract (2 teaspoons)

Instructions

- Preheat your oven to 400 degrees.

- Mix butter, flour, and sugar together.
- Then add the vanilla and almond extract as well as the eggs. Use a hand mixer on low speed or a spoon to mix the ingredients together.
- Scoop cookie batter onto an ungreased baking sheet.
- Bake for about 8 minutes.
- Allow to cool before you serve.

Nutritional facts:

Calories. 172

Carbohydrates.   26 g

Phosphorus.   22 mg

Potassium. 29 mg

Protein.   2 g

Sodium   56 mg

Lemon cake

Prep time – 10 min

Cook time – 1 hour 30 min

Total time – 1 hour 40 min

Ingredients

(24 servings)

- Butter (2 cups)
- Powdered sugar (4 cups)
- Grated lemon zest (2 teaspoons)
- Lemon extract (1 teaspoon)
- Eggs (6)
- Sifted all-purpose flour (3 ½ cups)

Instructions

- Preheat your oven to 350 degrees.
- Cream butter on low speed with an electric mixer until light and fluffy.
- Slowly add in sugar and lemon zest; mix thoroughly.
- Add lemon extract and the eggs, one at a time, mixing after each addition.
- Add flour gradually and mix well.
- Pour batter into a greased and floured pan
- Bake for one hour, 20 minutes. You will know it is done when a toothpick inserted in the center of the cake comes out clean.

Nutritional facts:

Calories.   279

Carbohydrates.   34 g

Phosphorus.   139 mg

Potassium.   108 mg

Protein.   10 g

Sodium.   127 mg

Whipped Cream Pound Cake

Ingredients

(30 slices)

- Butter or margarine - 2 sticks (softened)
- Eggs (6)
- Sugar - 3 cups
- whipping cream (½ pint)
- cake flour - 3 cups (sift once before you measure)
- Vanilla   flavoring (1 teaspoon)

Instructions

- Preheat your oven to 350 degrees.
- Oil and flour a tube/ baking pan.
- Ensure that all ingredients are at room temperature.

- Mix sugar and margarine together until fluffy.
- Then add the eggs, one at a time, beat before you add the next one.
- Slowly add the whipping cream and flour, mixing between each addition.
- Beat mixture for approximately 30 seconds, then stir- in the vanilla flavoring.
- Pour the batter into your greased and floured tube pan; bake for 60 minutes.

Nutritional facts:

Calories. 249

Carbohydrates.   35 g

Phosphorus.   24 mg

Potassium.   120 mg

Protein.   8 g

Sodium   192 mg

Fruit Crunch

Ingredients

(8 servings)

- Tart apples - 4 (pare, core and slice)

- Sugar (¾ cup)

- Sifted all-purpose flour (½ cup)

- margarine - 1/3 cup (Softened)

- Rolled oats (¾ cup)

- Nutmeg (¾ teaspoon)

Instructions

- Preheat your oven to 375 degrees.

- Place the apples in a greased square 8-inch pan.

- Mix the other ingredients in a medium-sized bowl and spread the mixture over the apple.

- Bake for approximately 35 minutes or until the Apple turns lightly brown and tender.

Nutritional facts:

Calories   217

Carbohydrates.   36 g

Phosphorus.   37 mg

Potassium. 68 mg

Protein.   1.4 g

Sodium.   62 mg

Sunshine Salad

Prep Time: 10 Mins

Ingredients

(9 servings

- Lemon -flavored gelatin (3 ounces/ 1 package)
- Crushed pineapple – 1 can with its own juice
- Boiling water (1 cup)
- Cold water (½ cup)
- Medium Carrots - 2
- Salt (1/8 tablespoon)
- Mayonnaise (for topping)

Instructions

- Pour the contents of the gelatin packet into a bowl.
- Add boiling water and stir until gelatin completely dissolves.
- Add cold water and stir. Add salt and crushed pineapple.
- Keep the mixture in the refrigerator until the gelatin begins to thicken.
- Peel the carrots, then grate.

- Add the carrots to the mixture and stir
- Pour the mixture into a square pan and refrigerate until it's firm.
- Then cut into square shapes and serve on crisp lettuce leaves.
- Use the mayonnaise as a topping

Nutritional facts :

Calories. 61

Carbohydrates. 15

Dietary fibers.   1 g

Phosphorus.   25 mg

Potassium.   119 mg

Protein. 1g

Sodium.   64 mg

Cherry Shortbread

Prep time – 30 min

Cook time – 20 min

Total time – 50 min

Ingredients

(20 servings)

- unsalted butter – 4 ounces
- plain flour (180 g/ 6-ounces)
- caster sugar – 2 ounces
- glazed cherries - 2 tablespoons (chopped)

Instruction:

- Preheat your oven to 190 degrees.
- Mix the butter and the sugar together until the texture is smooth.
- Add in flour and stir to give a smooth paste.
- If using cherries, add them now and stir gently.
- Gently roll out the mixture on a work top/ surface until the paste is half-inch thick.
- Cut into desired shape and place on an oiled baking tray.
- Sprinkle the caster sugar over the shapes and refrigerate for approximately 20 minutes.
- Bake in the preheated oven for 20 minutes or until it turns golden brown.
- Keep aside to cool.

Nutritional facts:

Calories. 190

Carbohydrate.   4.5g

Dietary Fiber Sugars. 12g

Protein. 2 g

Plain Scones

Ingredients

Makes 8-12

- self-raising flour (225 g)
- butter (55 g)
- a pinch of salt
- caster sugar (25 g)
- milk (150 ml)
- One egg, beaten to glaze, you could use milk as an alternative

Instruction:

- Heat your oven to 220 degrees.
- Grease your baking sheet.
- Mix the salt and flour together then rub in the butter.
- Add sugar and milk to get a soft dough.
- Place the dough on a floured work surface and knead gently.
- Spread the dough then use a cookie cutter to cut out round pieces. Repeat the step till you cut out all the dough. Place them on a baking sheet.

- Use a brush to apply the beaten egg on the top of the scones.

- Glaze the top of the scones with the beaten egg.

- Bake for 15 minutes until the scones are golden brown.

Conclusion

People with kidney disease need to reduce their intake of sodium, phosphorus, and potassium to make it easy to manage the disease. This book has compiled a list of all the high-phosphorus, potassium, and sodium foods that you should avoid or limit if treating kidney disease.

Your dietary restrictions and the recommended nutrient intake varies depending on the stage of your kidney disease. While it may seem like the renal diet is restrictive, there are still several options of delicious foods that are well-balanced, healthy, and are kidney-friendly. It may seem daunting to succeed in a renal diet, but with the help of a renal dietitian and your healthcare provider, you can design a renal diet that will suit your personal needs.

Other Books by the Author

- CELIAC/ COELIAC DISEASE AND THE GLUTEN-FREE DIET: The Adult and Children's Guide to Live Pain-Free. https://amzn.to/2O2b8MP

- HERBAL MEDICINE. The Beginner's Guide: Natural Remedies for Healing Common Ailments with Medicinal Herbs https://amzn.to/2t0VB8w

- THE GALLBLADDER DIET: Foods to Eat, Causes, Diagnosis, Tips for Recovery & Prevention and Natural Remedies to Cure Gallstones without Surgery https://amzn.to/313cTi6

- CELERY JUICE: The Natural Medicine for Healing Your Body and Weight Loss (Contains Secret Celery Recipes) https://amzn.to/2tTiISQ

- ALKALINE PLANT-BASED DIET FOR BEGINNERS: Your Complete Guide for Weight Loss, Boost Your Energy, and Cleanse Your Body with the Alkaline Diet. https://amzn.to/3aPZrSX

- LOW CALORIES DIET PLAN: Foods to Eat to Lose Weight and Stay Healthy. Includes 1,200 to 1,700-Calorie Meal Plans https://amzn.to/37vVyk1

- THE DIVERTICULITIS GUIDE TO LIVE PAIN-FREE: Diverticulitis Diet Plan, Foods to Eat & Avoid, Diagnosis and Tips for Causes, Recovery and Prevention https://amzn.to/38HTu8U